HEAR AGAIN

Back to Life with a Cochlear Implant

by Arlene Romoff

LEAGUE
FOR THE HARD OF
HEARING
PUBLICATIONS

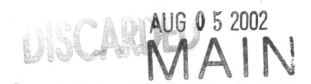

League for the Hard of Hearing Publications
71 West 23rd Street
New York, NY 10010

Library of Congress Cataloging-in-Publication Data

Romoff, Arlene
Hear Again: Back to Life with a Cochlear Implant

p. cm

Includes index
ISBN 0967784301

1. Hearing Impaired   2. Cochlear Implants
I Title

RF 681.7 693M33 1999

This book is published by the League for the Hard of Hearing. Since 1910, the League has provided comprehensive services to people who are deaf and hard of hearing, and has educated the public about hearing loss. Its services for children and adults with cochlear implants include a National Adult Cochlear Implant Rehabilitation Center, a Cochlear Implant Training Institute, an Adult Cochlear Implant Support Group, and programs which offer diagnosis, evaluation, counseling, rehabilitation, consultation and training.

Editor: Karin Mango
Photography: Vincent Amesee
Design: Tribich Design Associates, Inc.

For my husband, Ira,
and my children, Michael and Emily

ACKNOWLEDGEMENTS

This book would not have been possible without the encouragement and support of many wonderful people and the amazing technology of email, linking us together. Rather than try to compile a very long list of names, where I would surely overlook someone inadvertently, I will simply thank everyone who took the time to email their thoughts and insights to me. I treasured every message, and each one has helped shape this volume.

I also extend my heartfelt thanks to:

• My surgeon, Dr. Ronald Hoffman, and my audiologist, Betsy Bromberg, whose expertise and skills enabled me to have a miracle to write about.

• The wonderful people at the League for the Hard of Hearing, for more reasons than I can list here; that would be another book. I am grateful to Keith Muller, Executive Director, and Joe Brown, Director of Development, for their encouragement and assistance in producing this book.

• Peter Constantinidis, for maintaining the CI Forum, the email bulletin board that enabled my CI updates to reach so many people. "The Forum" allowed me to communicate with people literally from all over the world. Their comments, stories, and words of encouragement were inspirational.

• All those whom I've quoted on these pages. Some I've known a long time, some briefly, and some I've only met through email communications: Beth Agin, Sam Agin, Ronnie Armel, Joan Baras, Sharon Bell, Linda Benton, Lisa Carling, Izzy Cohen, Phylisse Cook, Julie Culver, Nancy Delaney, Cindy Floyd, Rachel Friedland, Bryna Gamson, Dave Gibb, Carolyn Ginsburg, Carol Granaldi, Trudy Green, Lise Hamlin, Greg Heller, Richard Herring, Jan Honig, Jane Hye, Ginny Jermanok, Judy Jonas, Bernard Klein, Nancy Kingsley, Anne-Marie Liss, Janet

McKenna, Jonathan Miller, Sue Miller, Keith Muller, Emily Romoff, Michael Romoff, Alice Rosenblatt, Pat Tomlinson, Janet Traub, Rudy Vener and Mardie Younglof. Every effort has been made to obtain permission for each reference, but this has not always been possible.

- My friends from Advocates for Better Communication (a.b.c.), the Costume Restoration Group, European American Bank (EAB), Eastern Association of Equipment Lessors (EAEL), N.J. Arts Access Task Force, N.J. Division of the Deaf and Hard of Hearing Advisory Council, Self Help for Hard of Hearing People (SHHH), my speechreading classes, and Temple Beth Or — who will recognize themselves on these pages. My life is richer for knowing you all.

- Karin Mango, not only for her editing expertise, but also for the pleasure of working together.

- Jay Tribich, for the fine design of this book, and for his insights and valuable suggestions.

- Doug Lynch, Manager of Marketing Communications at Advanced Bionics Corporation, for supplying the diagram of the Clarion cochlear implant device pictured in this book.

This book would not have been possible at all without the love and steadfast devotion of my husband, Ira. I am also touched by the interest and assistance of my children, Michael and Emily, who I am getting to know so much better, now that I can hear again.

PREFACE

What a great pleasure it's been to read Arlene Romoff's *Hear Again*! Not only because it's the story of a great triumph over a frightening disability, but because Arlene's perspicacity, sensitivity, and shining good humor come through on each page.

We found, as you read it, that doors of your perception open, making you realize just how important that often forgotten sense of hearing really is.

Enjoy this book, as we did, and expect to be surprised at every turn of the page.

Karen and Gene Wilder

In 1989 Karen Webb, speech language pathologist and then Director of Adult Communication Therapy at the League, coached Gene Wilder for his role as a deaf man in the movie "Hear No Evil, See No Evil." Subsequently Gene helped develop, and appeared in, the League's speechreading videotapes, "I See What You're Saying," which have been distributed nationally. The Wilders were married in 1991 and have continued to be committed to the League's work.

"Those who sow with tears shall reap with joy."
— Psalms 126:5

IN THE BEGINNING . . .

I never intended to write a book — but then again, I never intended to lose all of my hearing either. I wasn't born that way. I had normal hearing until I was about 20 years old — and then, the slow descent into deafness began. There was never any cause found for my drop in hearing — no trauma, no illness. It was diagnosed as a sensorineural hearing loss, for which there is no known cure. Little by little, slowly but surely, my hearing kept declining until, 30 years later, I had virtually none.

Trying to function with less and less hearing was emotionally exhausting. I struggled constantly to keep up with the skills I needed to cope with this unstoppable process. No sooner had I found the right hearing aids and perfected the needed lipreading skills, I would lose more hearing, requiring different electronics and even more coping skills. It was a constant game of catch-up that I was always destined to lose.

I had a James Bond assortment of assistive devices, not just hearing aids. I used amplified phones, personal FM and infrared systems, text telephones (TTY's), telephone Relay services, captioned televisions, plus lipreading classes. You name it, I found it and used it! One device that kept me functioning long after I ever could have with hearing aids alone, was my auxiliary microphone, a little gizmo that attached right onto my hearing aid by a connecting wire and plug. I would hold the cigarette-sized microphone right up to a person's mouth "interview-style" so that I would get as much usable speech sound as I could to help me lipread the rest.

I had always said that when my auxiliary mic no longer worked for me, that's when I would get a cochlear implant. I knew that day would eventually arrive. I just didn't know when.

In the same way that people remember where they were on the day Kennedy was shot or when the astronauts landed on the moon, I remember exactly when my auxiliary mic stopped working for me. It was that traumatic. We had gone out to dinner with another couple, friends of ours. I had always given my auxiliary mic to the person next to me, so at least I could have a one-on-one conversation with somebody. As we started to chat — the same way I had done countless times before — I noticed that my auxiliary mic wasn't bringing in any usable sound. Where was the sound? The auxiliary mic wasn't broken — I could tell it was on — but I couldn't hear my friend. Intellectually, I knew this moment would arrive. I had, after all, been losing my hearing for almost 30 years, so there had to be an end some-time. The logic of that theory was inescapable, but the emotions were some-thing else again. This was the moment I had anticipated for so long. The jig was up — finally.

I had already met people who had gotten cochlear implants, so the technology was not totally foreign to me. Actually, it was more of a hope-ful situation than a depressing one. This was the last and ultimate gadget in my "bag of tricks" that I had resorted to during my entire hearing loss odyssey. The cochlear implant was my last hope at functioning effectively in the world as I knew it — my hearing world.

Most of my friends and family had never even heard of cochlear implants. They have asked me how I knew about them. "How could I not have known about them?" I would always reply. I had researched every pos-sibility that would help me hear. I knew that although the whole idea of cochlear implants sounded futuristic, the future was here and now.

One doesn't just walk into a doctor's office and order a cochlear implant. I had to be evaluated first with a series of audiological and medical tests. Two things had to be determined, basically: was my hearing poor enough and was the physiology of my ears normal enough? I passed both bat-teries of tests with flying colors. In this topsy-turvy situation, doing poorly on the hearing tests was good because that meant that I would qualify as a candidate for the implant. If I heard too well, that would be bad. For once, I was happy to have "failed" a hearing test.

Once I was declared a candidate, the surgery date was set. I had to decide which ear I wanted to have implanted. Since the hearing in the implanted ear is usually destroyed, I didn't want to give up my better ear even though it heard so poorly. I preferred to use my left ear, which was vir-tually "dead." Another test, called a "prom stim," was performed to see if the auditory nerve in that ear could be stimulated. Much to my relief, the auditory nerve was very much alive, so I stayed with my decision to implant my worse ear.

I then had to choose between the two FDA-approved devices that were currently available. In a process similar to deciding which refrigerator to buy, I researched my options and decided on the Clarion S-Series Cochlear Implant made by Advanced Bionics Corp.

There are two components to the cochlear implant, internal and external. (See pages 248-249.) The internal component, which has to be surgically implanted, consists of a computer chip, a magnet, and an electrode array. The computer chip and magnet are inserted under the scalp, and the electrode array is threaded into the cochlea of the ear. The surgery, which is not considered a difficult procedure, requires general anesthesia and an overnight stay in the hospital. About a month later, after the incision heals up, the external component is attached and activated.

The external component consists of a magnet and a microphone on a headpiece about the size of a quarter. The magnet holds the headpiece in place on the scalp. It is attached by a thin cord to the speech processor, a beeper-sized computer that translates the sounds picked up by the microphone on the headpiece. As technology continues to advance, the speech processor will be miniaturized so that it will eventually fit behind the ear, similar in size to a hearing aid.

To explain briefly how this apparatus works: the sound is picked up by the microphone of the headpiece, then sent down the cord to the speech processor, where it is converted to a signal and sent back up the cord. It crosses through the scalp by radio waves. The internal computer chip receives the signal and sends the code over to the electrodes that are in the cochlea, telling them how and when to stimulate the auditory nerve. These electrodes stimulate the auditory nerve thousands of times per second. The auditory nerve then sends the signal to the brain, which perceives it as sound. If this sounds miraculous, then you're getting the right picture!

As for my surgery, it all went according to plan — more or less. Anesthesia tends to make me very nauseous and jumpy, so I wasn't feeling too well afterward. The actual surgery went fine, and I had virtually no problems with the healing process. Whatever pain I had was relieved with Tylenol. Some people have temporary dizziness, but I didn't. Four weeks later, I was ready to get the external component. Getting "hooked up" is the term everyone uses.

A funny thing happened between the surgery and my Hookup Day. I received request upon request from friends, family and colleagues, to please let them know how I did when I got hooked up. I'm quite active doing advocacy work for people with hearing loss. (Although this would technically be considered "volunteer work," I prefer to say that I work for organizations that can't afford me.) Because of my involvement in this field, there were plenty of people other than my immediate family and friends — those with hearing loss and professionals in the field — who were keenly interested in learning about my cochlear implant experience.

Getting the word out wasn't difficult to do, having the Internet and email at my disposal. So on the first two days of my Hookup — Day 1 and Day 2 — I sent out the following emails to about 75 of my closest friends, family and associates. I also sent these emails to an Internet bulletin board devoted solely to cochlear implant issues, called the CI Forum, which reaches several hundred people worldwide. So, literally hundreds of people received these two messages:

December 1, 1997 — Day 1

I was hooked up to my Cochlear Implant (CI) external processor today and I know many of you wanted to know how I did — so here goes. My surgery was on October 29th and I am still healing up, but feeling pretty normal now.

First the headline — I DID GREAT! By the end of the very first programming session, I could understand random sentences spoken by the audiologist, without looking. In the car going home, I could understand my husband, Ira, without looking most of the time. I could also understand most of the weather report on the radio and some of the news. I return tomorrow for more programming, and then again in two weeks. For those who want a more detailed account, keep reading.

I received the Clarion S-series implant, the new internal component and external speech processor. Because the implant site on my scalp was still a bit swollen from the surgery a month ago, my audiologist, Betsy Bromberg, put a stronger magnet in the microphone/headpiece. She thought it would fall off a lot, but it has stayed on pretty well if I don't touch it at all. When the swelling goes down a bit, she thinks that she will be able to use a weaker magnet. The speech processor is about the size of a fat cigarette pack and is worn at waist level. The headpiece is brown to match my hair, and the wire, which attaches to the processor, is flesh-colored.

With the speech processor attached to the computer, she first set upper and lower volume levels for eight different pitches, which I guess were the eight electrode pairs in the internal component of my implant, the part in my head. After that, we tried to balance them so they all were at about the same volume level. She tested me to see if I could hear any sounds that she made while my eyes were closed. She then tested me to see if I could hear how many sounds she made, again with my eyes closed. Then she wrote down two-syllable words and said them while I looked at this list of words, and she asked me to repeat which words she said, without looking at her. She added a few more two-syllable words, which I also repeated without looking. She wrote down three sentences which I looked at, and I had to tell her which sentence she had said without looking at her. And then she said simple sentences, such as "what is your name," "where do you live," and I had to repeat them back without looking at her. After that, she said random sentences, like "I want a cup of coffee," and I had to repeat those back without looking at her. I got everything correct right away, except one of the last sentences, and I got all of that on the second try. I felt as if I had just run a marathon, and won! And my husband, Ira, was sitting there, watching it all with tears in his eyes.

The audiologist loaded my speech processor with three programs: the first was the basic one we started with, the second had the speech frequencies louder than the higher and lower frequencies, and the third program had the high frequencies louder. This was all using one speech strategy, the way the speech processor software interprets sounds. When I go back tomorrow, she will try a different speech processing strategy to see if there is any difference. That is how she prefers to do things, not too much on the first day.

The sound I am hearing is weird and electronic, but for some reason I can still understand a lot of speech through it. This type of sound is expected on the first day and it is supposed to change as I become more accustomed to the implant, and as the programming changes. It all seems a lot like a Moog synthesizer doing the talking — or R2D2, the robot. This is strange to have coming in, but the sound that I had been getting from my hearing aid was so horrendous that this is actually an improvement. With my hearing aid, all the sounds grated on my nerves — like running your fingernail over a blackboard — but these electronic sounds don't make me jump at all. And I have been so used to trying to figure out speech from garbage noise, that this isn't much different, except that I can actually understand some speech!

On the way home in the car, I could hear my husband, Ira, without looking, which is pretty incredible. Not everything, but most of what he said, I could tell without looking. Also, when we listened to the radio, I could understand most of the weather report and, sometimes, some of the news.

Two interesting things have already emerged. First, now that I hear myself — Oh, my gosh, I have a New Yawk accent! (I hadn't heard that in quite a while!) And the other thing was that when we were listening to the news on the radio, I asked Ira if the person reporting was a woman, and he said, "Yes it was." The last time I heard the news on the radio (about 25 years ago), there were no women doing the newscasts! I feel a little like Rip Van Winkle!

So for Day One, this is pretty astounding because everyone says that it will only get better and better. As far as I'm concerned, Day One already exceeded my expectations for the entire implant because all I modestly wanted was to hear a few more consonants to be able to lipread better. I got that already and much more!

Thank you all for your support and encouragement. It has really meant a lot to me, and you all have been wonderful.

December 2, 1997 — Day 2

I drove into the city for my second appointment with the audiologist, to be reprogrammed. (Programming the speech processor is called "mapping.") As I drove, I listened to the radio in the car, which certainly is a lot more interesting than driving along in the silence that I am used to (and get drowsy with). I was able to understand some of it, mostly the weather report. Numbers seem to come in quite clearly, and some of the news, and even some traffic advisories. A lot depended on who was speaking — some of it was just noise.

The audiologist went through the same procedure as the day before, finding the very lowest volumes that I could still hear and the volumes that I found the most comfortable for all the eight electrode pitches, from low to high. We then tried to equalize them in volume so that they were all about the same loudness, then we tried the basic program using those settings. The amount of power that this program gave me was about 20% stronger than the previous day. In other words, my auditory nerve could tolerate that much more sound than the day before. I don't know the exact implications of this, but from what I understand about this process, the more powerful the program, the more nuance of sound you can get with it, and ultimately perform better with it.

The audiologist then told me to close my eyes and try to repeat three complex sentences that she recited. She said she would help me if need be. A sample sentence was: "Meet me at the corner in front of the drugstore." I was able to understand all three sentences without looking, on the first try. I didn't hear all of the words exactly, but with the context, I was able to repeat them immediately. This was considered a really excellent response for just the second day.

Next, we tried a different programming strategy for the speech processor to see if that made any difference for me — better or worse. She couldn't get the volume levels up enough to program it in the optimum way, so she tried an alternative method which would sacrifice clarity, but the resulting program sounded awful, so we didn't save any of those programs.

I mentioned to her that when I played the piano at home, I was only hearing some of the highest treble notes, nothing below except weird electronic wails, so she made a program that boosted the bass. And the third program we saved boosted the trebles, which she said sometimes makes speech easier to understand.

I then drove to Ira's office. Being in an environment where there was background noise or other people talking was totally different than the absolute quiet I had just been tested in. There was a lot of electronic noise, and the sound of people's voices coming and going was still very electronic and weird.

We went to a cocktail party, unexpectedly, which I definitely wasn't prepared for, and that whole experience was just noise. I couldn't really understand anyone with all that noise. I have an auxiliary microphone for the CI — the sort that I used to use with my hearing aid — so I have to figure out how to work that into my repertoire and fiddle with all the settings. Music was nonexistent for me at this party, just loud electronic "wind," nothing melodious. It's anyone's guess if I will be able to hear music as music eventually.

There's still a huge adjustment period going on, with so much electronic noise coming in. So if anyone is going to see me in the next few weeks at holiday parties, meetings or social gatherings, they will have to please bear with me as I get used to this new contraption! It's got great possibilities, but it is a beast that has yet to be tamed.

A few highlights of Day 2:

Waiting for the elevator, I heard it "ding" so I knew which elevator car had arrived. I can't tell you how many elevators I've missed in the last few years, or how vigilantly I've had to scan the lights on banks of elevators to know when they've arrived.

I tried playing my favorite Chopin Nocturne on the piano, plus a few scales — and although it still sounds weird, the sound did seem to be following the melodic line, which didn't happen yesterday, so maybe there's hope that I might eventually hear it like a piano. The piano sounded better when I only played the melodic line, no accompaniment, and I could follow it better when I knew what it should sound like. I also played scales, and was able to hear some of the bass range of the piano, which I couldn't hear at all yesterday. (And all I could think of was, "AH, the revenge of my piano teachers! She's finally practicing her scales!")

My audiologist doesn't want me to try the telephone yet; she wants me to wait until I've had a week's experience with the CI. It is probably good advice for me since with all of this strange electronic sound, coping, and having expectations, it's very draining emotionally. Normally, she would have people wait two or three weeks before trying the phone, but since I had responded so quickly, she thought one week would be right for me.

I have another appointment in two weeks, and then three weeks after that. So the process seems to be a gradual adjustment and continual fine-tuning.

I was a bit overwhelmed by the responses I received. Stunned, in fact. I didn't realize that so many people not only were interested in my hearing odyssey, but were utterly fascinated by the whole topic! People wanted to know more — and more — and more. The comments were coming from hearing people, deaf people, almost-deaf people, and professionals. Here are some examples:

> "*It means so much to me to read your firsthand accounts with the implant. It gives me so much hope. As my hearing continues to get progressively worse (gradually), I know the implant is a very viable option. Thank you for taking the time to share all of this with us. Please keep me on your 'list' — I want to get every email about this.*"
>
> Carolyn G. (hard of hearing friend)

> "*I can't wait to hear about Day 2 and more, so keep the news coming!*"
>
> Laurie Hanin (Director of Audiology, League for the Hard of Hearing)

"Thanks for the updates. This process is so exciting and amazing to me. . . . It gives me hope that should I lose what I've got left, there's something to do about it."

Lise H. (hard of hearing friend)

"I can't wait to hear more about what the experience is like."

Michael Romoff (son)

"I love hearing your saga. Keep it coming. . . . Hope you don't mind but I've forwarded it to Jan Honig, the woman who runs the Fair Lawn Deaf Program with me. She's finding it fascinating too."

Judy Jonas (Deaf and Hard of Hearing professional)

"I've been fascinated by your last two emails . . . Please keep sending updates to let me know how you're doing. I'm thrilled for you and can't imagine what it must be like for you to hear things you have not been able to hear for years."

Alice R. (college friend)

"Reading these daily updates is truly a moving as well as an exciting and educational experience."

Keith Muller (Executive Director, League for the Hard of Hearing)

"Your detailed report is amazing and gives me an 'education' as to what a CI recipient may expect."

Richard Herring (Director, NJ Division of the Deaf and Hard of Hearing)

> **"** *Just read your Day 1 story and had tears in my eyes, even cried a bit. I am so happy for you . . . can't wait to hear [more].* **"**
>
> Ginny J. (friend)

> **"** *It is both wonderful and fascinating to share your journey back to hearing! . . . We breathlessly await the next installment! I am, by the way, forwarding your messages to [my son] Mike, who adores learning about your progress — as we all do. How wonderful for US to be part of your reawakening!* **"**
>
> Bryna G. (friend)

Hmmm, I thought. This is a little bit more than I expected. There were people responding who had similar hearing to mine who knew little or nothing about cochlear implants and what they could do. There were hearing professionals, some who worked with children, who were eager to learn as much as they could. How could I stop writing after just two days? I felt an obligation to continue. I figured that another few days should be enough, so I continued.

December 3, 1997 — Day 3

I went out for a walk today, just to see what I would hear outside in my usual itinerary around the neighborhood. I love to step on acorns to feel the crunch they make underfoot. With my CI, I discovered they make a "crunch" sound also! And kicking a pebble along with my foot also makes noise, and it sounded as it should. So did walking through leaves.

When I passed someone using a noisy leaf-blower, I didn't have to turn the volume down on my speech processor. With my hearing aid, I would have had to turn down the volume, or turn it off completely because it would have been much too loud to tolerate. With the CI, I just heard it as tolerable noise and I kept walking.

I also heard something which I couldn't identify, so I looked all around me, and when I looked up, I realized that it was an airplane flying overhead. My only experience with airplane noise in recent years was at the U.S. Tennis Open in Flushing Meadow where the planes (used to) take off right over your head and make a booming noise. I hadn't heard a high-flying airplane in quite some time.

The biggest change came when Ira came home from work. I thought I heard the door open and close (I was in another room), and then I heard him call my name! For years and years, whenever Ira came home, I would never hear him come in, and I would literally jump (!) when he either made a loud sound behind me or touched my shoulder from behind. Now he can call my name, and I'll hear him. Once we realized that I could respond to my name, we now have to undo the years of conditioning to touch my arm or wave a hand to get my attention. I know my children will like this a lot! They had gotten really good at getting my attention first — now they're going to have to practice saying "Mom."

I listened to the television, but that was mostly noise. I was able to follow some of the sound with the captioning, but it was still strange and electronic.

The sound of water running started to sound more as it should, and not just a loud electronic rush. This is interesting to me because people said that the robotic quality would start to diminish, and the brain would start to get accustomed to what it was hearing, and things would start to sound the way they "should." I had been a little doubtful about all this since so much still sounds so loud,

electronic and weird, but they say it all requires patience —
a quality I'm a little short on.

December 4, 1997 — Day 4

Your response to my CI chronicles has been both
heartwarming and encouraging. Your comments are fascinating to me as well. The most touching was from a friend
with a hearing loss who was surprised and happy to learn that
elevators "ding." She never knew it because she's never
heard it. So I will continue to report the day's doings. . . .

This is my fourth day since getting my CI, and it
was the first time that I had an inkling of things to come.
Everyone has told me that everything will get better, and
that the electronic noise will start to abate. Intellectually,
I believed them. Emotionally, I did not.

When I sat down to play the piano once again, I
could hear the lower register notes louder than the previous day. I had expected to hear them less electronic, which
was also the case a bit, but not louder. And when I say
louder, I mean that aside from manipulating the volume
control on the speech processor, I was just hearing *more*.
Reporting from day to day is a little difficult because the
changes are subtle, but there was definitely more sound
coming out of that piano. It still had an electronic quality,
but when one note was sounded at a time, I could follow
the melody. Playing everything together was still a jumble
beneath the melody line.

But while I was playing the piano, I heard a new
noise, and since it came again, I wondered — the telephone? Hearing it from another room? So I ran to the
kitchen, and it was the telephone ringing! I hadn't heard
that the day before; the sound was too muffled to really
identify it as the phone. But on Day 4, I could definitely

hear the phone ringing, because it rang at other times throughout the day, and I heard it each time, no matter where I was in the house. (No, I didn't pick it up — not ready yet! I left it to my answering machine to deal with.)

And another surprise happened. I heard another noise, sort of a chiming sound, but it didn't repeat. Could it be the doorbell? It was the beginning of the month, the time the gas meter reader usually comes, so I took a look out the window — and there he was, the meter reader at the door! I really didn't want to deal with gas meter readers at that point, so I just let him go on his way.

Later in the day, I heard the same sound. "Ah," I thought, "the doorbell again!" But when I ran to the window to see who was there — nobody! Okay, so I heard it wrong. But then I saw a UPS truck driving away, so I opened my door. Lo and behold, there was a package left on the front step. So it *was* the doorbell! Two for two!

I should mention that I usually have an alerting device for the phone, the doorbell and the fire alarm. But the antenna had broken off and I had to send it out for repair, so it was just me and my CI to help hear these sounds.

Now my curiosity was piqued, and for the first time since hookup, I really wanted to see what else I could hear, so I got in my car and headed for the supermarket. I hadn't been there since my hookup. (We've been eating out a lot, and bringing in even more!)

Taking out my car keys, I love the way they jingle! Car keys haven't jingled in a very long time, and today they really jingled. I can remember the exact day several years ago, when I stood on this exact same spot, and the car keys refused to jingle. I remember shaking them and shaking them, and turning up my hearing aid, but the jingle was gone. My keys had stopped jingling. With my CI, those keys jingle again. I know this may sound silly, but that sound was a benchmark in my hearing loss — a day that I could point to when I couldn't hear something anymore. So hearing those keys may seem trivial, but it means that sounds are coming back. For 27 years, things have been gradually going away, and now they are starting to return.

Now, back to the car . . . On the way to the super-market, I turned on the radio, curious to see if it sounded any different from the previous day. I tuned in to CBS AM Radio 88 — the music on the other stations is still just an electronic blur. The weather seems to be the easiest to understand, but I did seem to get more of the news, depend-ing on who was speaking. I could follow men's voices pretty well, getting phrases, enough to tell what they were talking about. But I did notice that I could understand some of the women's voices, which were only noise the day before. Some of it was still just noise, or incomprehensible. What is curious is that numbers come in very well. They keep announcing the time and all sorts of phone numbers to call for I have no idea what. Hearing numbers is a real novelty because when I first started to lose my hearing, the numbers were the first to go. I hadn't heard phone numbers in an age!

Once in the supermarket, I literally felt as if I had landed on an alien planet. The shopping cart wheels squawked, tearing off the plastic bag in the produce section whooshed, and I secretly suspect that some of those vents up in the ceiling are really speakers. I have no idea what they were playing, but it seemed that every time I heard a strange noise and no one was around me, I was under one of those "vents." I met a neighbor I hadn't seen in years, and we exchanged pleasantries — nothing dramatic, except for the fact that I did hear her voice.

In the evening, I arranged to meet Ira at the mall to pick up a few things. I soon discovered that the mall is a noisy place! I wasn't overwhelmed with sound — it was just noisy, and still quite electronic-sounding. I could field

Ira's voice, and as he was walking up ahead, he called my name to get my attention, and I heard him without looking! We both grinned! He called my name again later, and I turned around again. Yes, this could definitely be useful.

As every hard of hearing person knows, not being able to hear your name is a real nuisance. It comes up time and again — doctor's offices, motor vehicles bureau, etc., etc. No matter how much you remind people, they either forget or don't realize that you *really* can't hear your name being called. I thought immediately of the time, many years ago, when I was in a toy store, returning a gift. When I discovered that the salesperson had been calling my name, I told her that I just didn't hear her. She told me that she thought that I was spaced out on drugs or something.

Yes, I think I'm going to like being able to hear my name.

Another little surprise happened as we were strolling through a gift shop. I heard bells, and I realized that the clocks on the wall were chiming. This store had some electronic Westminster-type clocks, and when you pushed some buttons, the chimes would sound. When I got up close, they really sounded like chimes — not electronic! Since they were playing one tone at a time, I could hear them like real chimes, with pitches. What a surprise! I was like a little kid in a toy store, pushing all the buttons, trying out my new hearing. I could hear clock chimes!

And back home, we watched television again, and this time, I was able to follow the dialogue of a documentary with the captions. It was narrated by a British gentleman with a low-pitched voice, and I could hear him well enough to know that he had a British accent (something I would prefer to have, but oh, well!).

And the last item on my agenda for the day was to try out the auxiliary microphone that came with my speech processor. Like the auxiliary microphone I had used with my hearing aid, it is helpful in noisy surroundings. We are going to be attending a dinner in a noisy restaurant in a few days, and I wanted to have a "dry run" with this microphone before putting it into service. So I asked Ira to turn up the volume of the television while I hooked up the microphone, turning down the sensitivity setting and turning up the volume control on my speech processor. When Ira spoke, I heard him really well! I didn't hear the tv, and Ira said it was blaring! That looks promising! I'm now ready for my mic debut in a noisy environment.

Day 4 had been such an adventure and, for the first time, I felt that I was starting to experience this "it will get better" phenomenon that everyone had promised. So instead of wondering if this CI will really work, I'm looking forward to the changes tomorrow will bring.

After sending out those two updates, I received a flood of comments like these:

> **"**I cannot TELL you how interesting your updates are to me. Although I know something about CI's, I have never had an idea of how it really 'feels,' 'sounds,' and is. Thank you for your wonderful travelogue through your experiences!!**"**
>
> Pat Tomlinson (Deaf and Hard of Hearing professional)
>
> **"** **"**
>   more
>
> Laurie Hanin (Director of Audiology, League for the Hard of Hearing)

(Yes, that's all she wrote. I got the message!)

"We're delighted to read your saga! I have forwarded all four days of your progress to [my friend], who is deaf/blind. . . . He has just thanked me for forwarding your chronicles. My eyes tear . . ."

Carol G. (hard of hearing friend)

"Your letters are such a delight to read — they make me stop and listen and realize just how much I take for granted every day of my life."

Julie C. (my daughter's friend)

"Thank you so very much for sharing your heartwarming experiences. I look forward to reading more. I'm forwarding your emails to a friend of mine in Buffalo who is seriously considering a CI. Your experience will be an inspiration to her, I'm sure."

Sue M. (hard of hearing friend)

"Wow, makes me feel so positive if that time ever happens to me, I'm going to get the CI. . . . I'm proud of you and think you should keep on writing . . ."

Ronnie A. (hard of hearing friend)

"Carol G. forwarded your CI Chronicles to me. . . .Would it be okay with you if I forwarded [them] to a friend of a friend, who is losing more and more of her hearing?"

Jane Hye (Deaf and Hard of Hearing professional)

> **"** *I am sending a copy of your story to my hard of hearing aunt who is anxiously awaiting it.* **"**
>
> Sharon B. *(friend)*

I never imagined that what I wrote would have such an impact, and I knew that this was just the beginning of my story. It had always been my philosophy to have something good come from the ordeal of my hearing loss, the classic "when life gives you lemons, make some lemonade" outlook. That's why I had become so involved with advocacy for deaf and hard of hearing people. With comments like these now coming in, how could I stop writing? For the next year, I chronicled my experiences with my cochlear implant. As I continued to send updates on my progress, many people wrote encouraging me to publish this material so that others could benefit. This book is the result.

Bear in mind as you spend the next year with me, that I am a late-deafened adult. The way I function with my cochlear implant is directly related to my own hearing history. Since I once had normal hearing, my experience is different from those who have never heard sound, those who have always had a hearing loss or those who have been deaf for a long time. I don't want to discourage anyone from pursuing a cochlear implant for themselves; I just want to point out that the adaptation process is unique to each person.

I also want you to be aware that this is no ordinary diary of daily events. We're talking miracles here, true miracles of biblical proportions — allowing the deaf to hear. It's a humbling experience, and tends to make everyday complaints and nuisances seem trivial. This may account for my lack of anger or negative emotions. I mention this now because I may be faulted for sounding too happy, too joyful or painting too rosy a picture. The truth is that I am in absolute awe of being able to hear again. I don't think anyone can fully comprehend, unless they've experienced it themselves, what it is like to return to a world full of sound. I think you'll understand a little better as you journey through these pages. Join me now as my hearing odyssey continues.

THE CHRONICLES CONTINUE . . .

DAY 6
DECEMBER 6

I'm beginning to get used to the CI apparatus and the logistics of putting it on and taking it off. It's becoming part of me and the world is starting to sound very quiet without it. I used to enjoy the quiet without my hearing aid on, a respite from the harsh sound it was delivering to my ear. But I don't seem to have that feeling with the CI, even though there are a lot of strange and often weird sounds coming in. I can't wait to put it on in the morning to see what things will sound like today since I know they will most likely be different and possibly better, even if only slightly, from yesterday.

I had the chance to speak with someone yesterday who had always been tremendously difficult for me to understand, almost impossible in fact. She has a heavy Spanish accent, and our communication had dwindled to constant repetition, spelling out words, and even writing down words when necessary. Yesterday, I spoke with her in my house, in quiet, one-on-one, and I never asked her to repeat at all! I still had to look at her, but I could actually hear her voice. Although voices are still electronic in tone, they are starting to sound a little less so. I could also detect some of the nuance in her speech. I had grown accustomed to assuming that I was getting all the nuance of conversation from facial expression and body language, but now I realized that there was a lilt in her voice — and she has a very dynamic personality — so I was detecting subtleties in her speech that I had been missing before. "Delighted" is an understatement to describe her reaction at finally being able to communicate easily with me. We've only known each other a year and she has had so much patience in communicating with me. She got the rewards for her efforts yesterday — she did not have to struggle to talk to me.

I'm starting to get used to the idea that I can hear the phone ring. I even heard my fax line phone from another room, so I knew some faxes were coming in. It makes life a little more efficient, I guess.

The doorbell is also coming in fine. I have to mention that I have four very loud doorbells in my house, vestiges of the days when I could still hear them. Instead of just a "noise," I could actually hear a bell-like tone yesterday. This time, I didn't even look out the window to see if anyone was there. I ran right to the door and opened it. NO ONE WAS THERE, but now as an experienced doorbell-answerer, I looked for a package on the front step. Yes, the hit-and-run UPS driver had struck again!

The big event for the day was a dinner party, and I was going to be trying out my auxiliary mic for the first time, so that I could function in noise. I'm no novice with auxiliary mics because I have relied on them for the past few years with my hearing aid. They enabled me to function very well in noisy places. But using the mic requires planning, figuring out how you want to use it and where you want to put it. You can clip it right on to yourself, hold it "interview-style," place it on a table or clip it to the person you are talking to. It all depends on the situation.

In planning for this particular evening, I decided that since it was a sit-down dinner, I would just leave it clipped to my own clothing and turn to the person I wanted to hear. I figured I could always unclip it and go "interview" mode if need be. Having made that decision, I resolved to out-fit myself as elegantly as possible.

There's very little visible with a CI. The cord running down from the headpiece, under one's clothing to the speech processor clipped on at the waist, doesn't really show much — just the cord peeking out between the nape and the collar. But the wire from the auxiliary mic can be quite visible unless you choose your clothing carefully. By plugging into the speech processor and running the wire up under my clothing, I can clip on the auxiliary mic between the front buttonholes. Since the auxiliary mic is black, it's less conspicuous on darker clothing. If anyone starts wondering why all of a sudden I'm tending to wear dark clothing that buttons in the front, you'll know why! If I wanted to hold the mic "interview-style," I would have to pull the wires out from under the clothing and use its full length.

Yes, vanity does come into play here. If I had just clipped the auxiliary mic onto the outside of my clothing, I would have been more flexible. But with the wires from the processor and the wire from the auxiliary mic, at least for this occasion, I really didn't want to look (or feel) as if I were about to detonate!

In the car going into the city, I could understand Ira without looking — pretty neat! Once in the restaurant, I fiddled with the settings, having gotten the advice that turning the sensitivity down and the volume up would work best in noise. With a round table full of people, this was going to be a challenge, since I had no idea what I would be hearing, or if I would understand anything at all. Expectations — I'm not sure if I had any!

Strangely, with the CI set with the sensitivity down, along with the auxiliary mic, I didn't pull in any background noise. I was surprised to learn that there was guitar music playing, plus the general hum of a restaurant. I didn't hear it, nor did I want to. There's no doubt that if this dinner had been a week ago, with only my hearing aid, it would have been impossibly difficult. I would have tried to lipread, but I know I would have had to rely on Ira to be my oral interpreter.

I should explain that a bit, and introduce you to my husband. When Ira and I were married, I had normal hearing. As I lost my hearing, he was by my side, helping, every step of the way. I've come to learn that not all spouses are so supportive, so I consider myself very fortunate. Ira would scout for the best doctors, devices, anything that could possibly help me. In social situations, we had an unspoken way of communicating that indicated if I needed some assistance. I'm not even sure what we did — an eyebrow moving upward, a quizzical look — whatever — he would keep me included in the conversation by mouthing to me what was going on. If anyone had told me that I would eventually be able to lipread my husband without the benefit of sound, I would have said that was ridiculous! But, that's what happened as my hearing loss reached the profound level. Ira would oral interpret for me, mouthing the words, anything that I missed in conversation. And he would do it in such a natural manner that it wasn't very obvious to others. It was hard work for both of us, so to be relieved of this chore would certainly make social situations more enjoyable.

At our dinner table, I could hear some people clearly, others not as well, and some not at all. With that kind of hearing, though, I didn't need an oral interpreter! I could actually understand one woman two seats away — a personal best! When the auxiliary mic fielded more than one voice, it seemed to cut down on all comprehension. I fiddled with the settings, and I must mention that the volume and sensitivity knobs on this CI have far more power than their counterparts on a hearing aid. Turning up the sensitivity setting even slightly dramatically increases the range of sound. And then adjusting the volume level, I could sense the potential of this system, even though at this stage, I was fielding so much incomprehensible noise.

I knew that if I had any real trouble hearing someone, I could take the auxiliary mic and simply hold it up to that person's mouth, as I had done in the past, and I don't think I would have had any trouble understanding them. I didn't do that because I was trying to follow a whole table of conversation. There was still plenty of strange noise, but I actually functioned better than I had with the same group of people last year.

Did I have fun? Not really — I was working too hard. Was I glad that I came? Yes, because I was able to socialize and speak to people. I also found out that this CI, with a little bit of experience, could work in noise. Would I have been happy to be there using only my hearing aid? Absolutely not! Social situations had become far too difficult, so difficult, in fact, that I had begun to avoid them. I just couldn't function effectively with my hearing aid anymore.

With this experience, I now look forward to similar dinners and parties in the holiday season ahead — like next week! Is it too optimistic to think that my hearing will be a little better by then? A novel development! For 27 years I have been conditioned to expect less and less, so even to think that I might do better next time, really now — if I wasn't experiencing it firsthand, I would have said "in your dreams!"

DAY 7
DECEMBER 7

My hearing aid had been sitting on my dresser since last Monday, the day I started using my CI speech processor. I'm convinced now that I will not use it anymore. Some people do use a hearing aid in their unimplanted ear, but I know I will not be one of them. I'll eventually donate this aid so that it can help someone else, but until then, I'll just store it. I opened the battery case to remove the battery so that the aid would not be damaged, and then I closed the battery case flap. *CLICK!* Click? The battery case clicks when you close it? I never knew that! I tried it again. *CLICK!* And again. *CLICK!* How could I have known this? And I have to chuckle because this little hearing aid, which has served me for so many years, just couldn't go silently into the night. It had to have its last hurrah! I closed the battery case one last time. *CLICK.*

I've made piano practice a daily routine now, and today there was definitely a difference. When I played more than one note at a time, I didn't set off an electronic roar. Everything still has a synthesizer quality, but as I played my Chopin Nocturne for the umpteenth time, I think I could detect the base accompaniment beneath the melody. I say "I think" because it is so subtle, I'm not even sure. I suppose I'll know more in the next few days.

I should mention that over the years, as my hearing declined, I continued to play the piano even though I heard less and less. As long as I play pieces that I know, my brain always seems to supply the missing sounds that

I can't hear. I jokingly call this playing by the "Beethoven Method" since Beethoven, who also went deaf, must have experienced something similar.

I got into the car to run some errands, and I flipped on the radio — CBS Newsradio 88. See? I even know what to call it now because that's the way they identify themselves on the station. I noticed immediately that I could hear some of the women's voices clearer, even understanding some of the words they were saying. One of the announcer's voices was very clear, a deep voice. I realized that I could listen to his voice without "working" to hear — and I knew from experience that when you don't have to "work" at listening, you can concentrate on the content. It's a subtle difference, but it comes into play especially when there are no visual cues, such as with a radio or telephone. If the brain is trying to understand the words, it can't concentrate fully on the content. Interestingly, when I turned on the radio, instinctively I still worried whether I would hear it as well as yesterday, still conditioned to expect less hearing rather than more. I heard more.

Running errands presents the problem of different hearing environments and knowing how to adjust the CI settings. I imagine this will eventually fall into place as one program (hopefully) becomes "general purpose." Until I get the hang of this, I figure I'll just fiddle with the settings when it's necessary or convenient, and not worry too much about it now.

I stopped at the library to get some cassette tapes. Children's books were recommended because the dialogue is usually slower than adult books. I also took out *Peter and the Wolf*, figuring that was a good selection because it had narration, music, and individual instruments playing. When I popped the cassette into my car's player, I heard "Side 2, Chapter 6 — 'The Chocolate Fever'." It wasn't *Peter and the Wolf*, that's for sure, but I heard it — clearly. They must have put the wrong cassette in the bag, but I continued to listen anyway. It was a deep male voice, narrating slowly and expressively, and I heard and understood the whole thing. I had planned to play it on a Walkman, plugging it directly into the speech processor. But being able to hear it in the car was a surprise that now opens up even more possibilities for avoiding drowsiness and boredom while driving.

We went to a diner for dinner and it was unusually quiet for a change. I didn't bring the auxiliary mic — I don't have my act together just yet. I haven't converted over my "equipment bag" to the CI paraphernalia. I fiddled with the settings on the speech processor, lowering the sensitivity level and adjusting the volume. I still heard the background noise, but I could pick up some of Ira's voice. With lipreading, we were able to converse easily. It probably was good practice to listen in noise. Normal ears naturally ignore background noise. It would be nice if my brain can be trained to do the same.

Watching television in the evening, I had trouble fielding the sound, so I tried the program in my speech processor that accentuated the high frequencies, and I heard better with it. This was a surprise to me because two days before, that program was not better. But considering that today I was able to understand some of the female radio announcers, I must have gained some ability to hear high frequency sound. Don't ask me how this works or why. I'm just glad that for some reason, adapting to a CI is an ever-expanding experience. Now I know to try programs even if they don't work well initially since evidently things are changing all the time. Just as I had expected, it's going to be a learning experience.

DAY 8
DECEMBER 8

I realize now that I may be painting a little rosier than reality picture of life with my new CI. While it is true that I am able to understand speech one-on-one in a quiet environment, we all know that this is not the typical hearing experience. It is a noisy world, and while I am getting much more sound and comprehension now, trying to deal with that noisy world, particularly at this early stage of adaptation, is especially trying and exhausting.

There are two control knobs on the speech processor, and the way they react to noise and sound often defies common sense or predictability. It is trial and error, with lots of trial and even more error. Dealing with this on a continual basis, constantly moving from one hearing situation to another, is bewildering and exhausting. My hearing seems to change slightly with each day and I don't have any idea where to put the settings for various situations — stores, outside/noisy, outside/quiet, social gatherings, background music, other people talking, group situations — plus combinations of the above. It is difficult to find the right settings, especially when the circumstances are fleeting. I imagine this will get better — how much better is an unknown. Comfort in noise becomes the priority, and then, hopefully, some sort of speech comprehension will get thrown in.

The highlight for yesterday was hearing on the phone! Ira and I spoke to each other using the two phone lines in our house. It became apparent that just by holding the receiver up to my CI headpiece produces clearer sound than the plug-on suction cup accessory that attaches to the phone. Since just holding the receiver up to the microphone on the head-piece was working, I didn't try to use the auxiliary mic or other plug-in gizmos that are available. I also had a successful call with my sister, who was delighted to be able to talk to me without Relay. (She hates Relay.) The call was far from perfect — she did have to repeat several times — but she said she was repeating less than she would have had to for a Relay operator!

Relay service, for those who are not familiar with it, allows people who use TTY's — the typing kind of telephone that displays printed text on a screen — to phone people who don't have this special equipment. It's essentially a three-way call, where the third party is the Relay operator who has a TTY. The Relay operator types whatever the hearing party says to the TTY user. The TTY user, in turn, can speak directly to the hearing party. I started using Relay about seven years ago when I could no longer function on a regular voice phone.

I am not in a hurry to use a regular voice phone all the time. Far too much emotional baggage is attached to phone use. With my fluctuating hearing loss, I have spent over 20 years struggling with the phone, so I do not want to struggle just to say I can use a voice phone. I have always advocated for hard of hearing people to use all options available to them to make their lives easier, and that means using Relay for phone calls that may be difficult to hear or that don't require that personal touch. So I'm not quite ready to go "public" just yet, not until I feel confident enough and have had enough experience with the receiver and the settings, and am able to understand a variety of voices. I will tell you, though, that I answered the phone today and fielded my first "junk call," a credit card solicitation. I got about half of it, and you know I didn't ask her to repeat!

We went to the theater last night to see a captioned performance at the Paper Mill Playhouse in Millburn, New Jersey. I used the infrared system as well, and I could hear some of the dialogue. I was able to use the same receiver that I had used with my hearing aid, connecting my speech processor to the receiver with a "patch cord." Infrared systems deliver the sound picked up by the stage microphones directly to the receiver worn by the audience member. It virtually eliminates the distance between the sound source and the receiver.

The show, *Children of Eden*, was good, but it was not the best type for a novice CI user. It was mostly singing and, surprisingly, some of it actually sort of sounded like singing, when there was no choral background. The problem I was encountering was that I really didn't know where to set anything — the CI or the infrared controls — and a lot of it came in very loud. I also don't know if the infrared was having problems, or my speech processor or me, because the sound kept changing volume as if something was loose. Later on, my hearing was getting louder and softer too, so I really didn't know what was wrong, and I was very concerned about it. I didn't know if the speech processor was damaged or what. In the morning, my speech processor seemed fine, but I called my audiologist and she said that it was possible for my hearing to get tired, especially after a long day of listening. She said if that happened again, just to turn off the speech processor and wait a half hour before starting it up again. This should calm things down with my hearing.

Oops, I forgot to mention that she called me back by regular voice phone, and we had a normal conversation even though I was pretty apprehensive about it. I used the volume control on the phone to adjust to her voice. With that experience, I imagine that any future communication between us will be by regular voice phone. My plan is to gradually move over to voice phone use, but, as I said, I'm in no rush.

Because of that sound overload, and knowing how taxing it is trying to cope with noisy environments at this stage of the game, I opted out of a holiday party this evening — too stressful right now. I've never copped out of social engagements because of my hearing, but since there are other social events cropping up very soon, I decided to be good to myself. No martyr here.

The highlight of the day was that for the very first time, driving home from the theater in the dark after the show, I was able to follow the conversation with the three other people in the car. I always had to sit there in bored silence because it's impossible to lipread in the dark or from behind. Flipping on lights and trying to turn around, especially after a long evening, was always too stressful, even if I could follow, which I probably couldn't. But last night, I was following somewhat, helped by the fact that the microphone for the CI is behind my ear, so I could pick up sound from the back seat without turning around.

And a few little surprises today too: I could understand most of what the clerk in the post office was explaining about the nuances of postal insurance rates. And I also heard the teller at the drive-through bank. Drive-through windows have always been a gamble because if there was ever a problem, I couldn't communicate through the speakers or phone receiver. It surprised me to hear some words instead of the squawks I had grown accustomed to.

Words instead of squawks — that pretty much sums up what this CI is all about.

DAY 10
DECEMBER 10

The tonality of the CI has started to change a bit; it's still electronic, and has started to take on a raspy, hoarse quality, but I'm still able to field speech with that sound. Quiet environments, and speech closest to me come in clearest. The further away, the more distorted the sound is, and the more I have to rely on visual cues and lipreading.

I've figured out how to get the best sound out of my piano. Turning the sensitivity down produces more of a piano-like quality and less of that electronic warp. I also noticed that I think I can hear two notes together without setting off too much electronic "wind." I figured that I'd pull out some simple Bach Minuets, which have only a melody line and a single bass line. This way, I can play real music, and have a better chance of hearing it. It's a mystery what I will eventually be able to hear though — it's still so early.

Now I know that I can use the phone, at least for some voices. Some of the telephones in my house are clearer than others. I'm not sure why. It might be either the phone itself or the line it's on. I'm still not certain where exactly to hold the receiver. I have to position it so it is covering the microphone on the headpiece. To adjust the volume, I've been turning the volume up on the phone itself. When I turn up the volume setting on the speech processor, it tends to distort the speech, so it's good that I have the volume control phones.

I've had conversations with family members, and I've even turned down the opportunity to buy timeshares at the Flagship Hotel in Atlantic

City! I noticed that on the lengthier calls, over 15 minutes, the volume starts to diminish. Maybe the nerve is getting tired, as my audiologist suggested yesterday. This happened when I was on the phone with my sister and my son, so is something to be aware of at this point.

I notice that the hearing people who have used Relay with me still are conditioned to expect the Relay operator to interact with them. They seem to have to make the bigger adjustment, to speak at a regular pace without having to be reminded to speak slower. I guess they got conditioned to my voice and associate it with Relay! I don't have to make that adjustment because using the Voice Carryover feature of Relay, I always spoke at a normal pace since the hearing party heard me directly. I have to admit, though, that when I heard a dog barking in the background, I expected "(dog barking)" to appear on the telephone screen! I should mention that I am using an Ultratec Uniphone telephone, which can be used as a regular voice phone with volume control, or as a TTY that can be easily used with the Voice Carryover feature of Relay. I'm also finding that Caller ID is still helpful, as it was when I couldn't hear on the phone, to either identify the caller, or to be able to call them back by Relay if necessary. Unfortunately, not all calls are identified by Caller ID.

I was able to retrieve messages from my voice mail. We used to have a regular tape answering machine, and I used to listen to the messages over and over again to try and figure out what was being said. When that became futile, we switched over to voice mail so that I could have a Relay operator retrieve my messages. But yesterday, when I saw the flashing light indicating that there were messages, I decided to try to retrieve the messages myself. I knew what the recorded prompting message was, having had it typed by Relay operators so often, so I was able to follow that. But I could also follow the "press one," "press this and that" instructions to retrieve my message. I made the message repeat, and repeat again, just to make sure I understood what was being said, and I heard enough to know how to save it also.

I'll have to get a lot more experience and practice with other voices before I'll have the confidence to use the phone again on a regular basis. All the memories of the bad experiences I've had with the phone come flooding back, particularly being hung up on when I was asking people to repeat so much. I know I would be able to handle those situations better now, since I know to ask for assistance and patience when need be. I'm just not anxious to have to do that yet.

DAY 12
DECEMBER 12

I had thought that I wouldn't be giving as many updates, figuring that things would simmer down and that I would have less to report on a regular basis. But part of what I wrote two days ago is already obsolete!

I had written that I was in no rush to use a voice phone, that I figured I would gradually move over from Relay to using a regular voice phone. But I have been getting my voice mail by myself, I have been answering the phone and calling friends and family by voice phone, all with good results. Not perfect, but really a lot better than I expected. So today, I had to make some "real" phone calls to people I didn't know and I was faced with the dilemma — voice or Relay. I'm not really an adventurer, preferring the tried and true to the unknown, but I just couldn't bring myself to dial into Relay to try and resolve a billing error. I could always bail out and call Relay if need be, so I plunged ahead. I got through a few voice message menus, and I actually got to speak to a real live person in the correct department. I was doing fine, getting through most of the call, when I just couldn't catch something the voice on the other end was saying. Automatically, I heard myself say, "I'm sorry, I'm hard of hearing. Could you please repeat that?" And he said, "Sure, no problem."

Let me explain this. I used to tell people I was hard of hearing when asking them to repeat or speak slower. With my degenerative hearing loss, just as soon as I had mastered the lipreading and coping skills necessary to function at a certain level of hearing, I lost more hearing, starting the process all over again. I never caught up. When my hearing loss reached the profound level, a few years ago, I had to change the "message" to "I'm sorry, my hearing is very poor, could you please . . ." With that phone call using my CI, where I was getting most of the conversation and needed some repetition, the "hard of hearing" message was the appropriate term to use again. By referring to myself now as "hard of hearing," I had turned back the clock and the description of my hearing loss. I was going in reverse and my reaction was instinctive. Not only that, when I was first losing my hearing, I didn't know that saying "I'm hard of hearing" worked so well to manage a situation like that. The "hard knocks" of having been hung up on had taught me that lesson. It had taken me years to figure this out, and even then, I still had a hard time getting those words through my lips, coming to terms with my hearing loss. This time around, I had "been there, done that," so while it may not always be easy, it cuts the problem down to size, and I think I can handle that. I know that Relay is still right there if I just don't feel like coping with it all.

So today, all my calls were regular voice calls. I only had one problem with a recorded message. I couldn't understand it at all, so I called into Relay to find out what it was. It was an answering machine, and the Relay operator said it was very hard to understand (but he understood it). Yes, I'm on the phone, but it is still a "work in progress."

The other thing I wrote two days ago was that the piano sounded best with the sensitivity setting turned way down. Today, I discovered that almost any sensitivity setting was okay. Only the highest sensitivity setting brought on the weird electronic response. Everything else sounded pretty much the same as the best setting two days ago. I leave it to the professionals to tell me what's happening. The piano sounded a little more piano-like, but with a husky electronic echo, still not real piano or music, but not the same as a few days ago.

Hearing in a cocktail party setting was fine (it's the busy Christmas season, lots of parties and dinners). By using the auxiliary mic and turning the sensitivity setting down, the background noise was blocked out, and I could field the voices close to me. Cocktail parties seem to have an advantage over sit-down dinners because the people I am talking to are usually right next to me, and not across a table. I noticed again, though, that after conversing with some people for awhile, longer than 10 minutes, the volume of their speech started to decrease. Boosting the volume on my CI didn't make things better. This was the same phenomenon I had noticed on lengthy phone calls. It may have been because of the noise in the background, the lateness of day (getting tired of listening), or my nerve not being able to carry the same voice signal for an extended length of time. I don't know if this will change later on.

I visited with friends yesterday, the "Sewing Ladies" that I had not seen since before my surgery. We are all volunteers, doing costume restoration at a local historic house, the Hermitage, in HoHoKus, New Jersey. (Its claim to fame, other than its Gothic Revival architecture and outstanding vintage costume collection, is that George Washington slept there and Aaron Burr was married there.) These lovely ladies don't have email, so the first thing that they asked me was, "Can you hear?" You can imagine their expressions when I smiled and said, "Yes!" Speaking with a group of six women was harder for me than a noisy cocktail party. One voice came in very well, the highest-pitched one. The others were less clear, but I could still understand them with lipreading. I had worked in the sewing room for several years with these women before getting my CI, and had reached the point where I could not participate in their lighthearted "quilting bee" banter. It had become very difficult for all of us because they didn't want to exclude me from conversation, yet communication had become such a struggle. Yesterday, I got a glimpse of the nature of the conversations that I had been missing over the years, and it was delightful! Stories about children, grandchildren, problems, joys. What a wonderful education I was getting about the people I had been sitting next to for so long!

Over the years, people with normal hearing would often tell me "it's not important" when I missed parts of conversations. Those segments would immediately become "most important" to me. Now I'm starting to learn that, yes, some of it really isn't important, but it's so much better to be able to decide that for myself.

I also had a few new revelations. Things make noise when you drop them! I'm not sure how clumsy I've been in the past, but this may explain how my glasses could end up under the kitchen table without my knowledge. I am curious to know, though, if hearing people can also hear the sound of a toothpick dropping on a wood floor. I dropped one by accident, and only noticed it when I heard a faint little pitter-patter. Am I supposed to be hearing that sort of sound or did the engineers get carried away with this bionic ear? And if not, why wouldn't/couldn't they in the future?

And something else: I don't know if this is true of people with normal hearing, but before I had my CI, whenever I yawned, it would cut down the volume on the sound coming in. This doesn't happen with my CI — the sound keeps coming in right through the yawn. An improvement on nature, perhaps?

And one other sound that intrigued me was the beep of the groceries going through the scanner at the supermarket. I never used to know, when they scanned six cans of tuna fish, if they had really rung up six. The readout on the cash register only blinks slightly if you ring up the same price repeatedly. Today I could tell just by listening. Another one of life's little mysteries solved by my CI.

DAY 16
DECEMBER 16

I had my mapping yesterday, my third one, two weeks after hook-up. I was curious about what changes would occur with the mapping since I knew that my hearing had started to adapt to the sounds coming through my speech processor. My daughter, Emily, is home from college, so she came with me to the session. She has always had great empathy for other people, her mother included. As my hearing loss progressed, she became my hearing helper, taking on tasks like answering the phone or making phone calls, or just intervening when she knew that I couldn't understand what was going on.

I should mention, by the way, that Sunday was the first time I had seen Emily since I got my speech processor, and I can't tell you what a difference it made! Communication had become very difficult between us (and not because of the typical teen/parent tensions). She has a high-pitched voice, and I had lost all of my high-frequency hearing, so any communication required almost total lipreading, which is not only difficult but exhausting as well. I had gotten into the habit of interrupting her and putting words in her mouth, a behavior that was an attempt to make conversation easier to understand, but that also hindered real communication. Yesterday, as we spent the day together, she had to repeat very little, and I felt so calm and eager to hear what she had to say. I just wonder what mother-daughter chitchat we had missed over the years. I hope we can make up for some of that now, even by phone.

The CI mapping followed the usual routine, finding the lowest threshold of sound that I could hear for each of the eight electrode pairs, and then the volume that I found most comfortable for the same series. My numbers hadn't changed that much — a little here and there — which surprised me, but my audiologist said that with the Clarion device, people who do well right from the start stabilize very quickly with their threshold and comfort levels. We developed three new programs. One was basically the same as the program I had preferred after two weeks with the speech processor, the one that had the high frequencies boosted. The second was what she called my "power" program, to be able to field low volume voices when I need to. I don't know when I will use that, but I guess I'll figure that out later. And the third program was flat, with neither high nor low frequencies boosted. We also tried to eliminate the raspy, hoarse, f-f-f-f-f sound quality that I was hearing. She fiddled with some settings, increasing and decreasing volumes, changing tone qualities and asking me which sounded better. We settled on a setting which seemed more natural to me and then she tested me on several sentences without looking. I was able to repeat all the sentences except for one word which she had to repeat once. I got the beginning of one sentence because of the context. She loaded the programs into the speech processor, we chatted a bit and then we were on our way.

I was a little surprised about this mapping session. I had envisioned great changes or programming breakthroughs, but I guess since I was already hearing on the phone and doing so well in general, there were no real problems to address or correct. This was just a tune-up, fine-tuning what my brain had already adapted to. And that seems to be the process. If the mapping is doing well enough to allow me to function so well so soon, then the progress will come from the brain's continuing to adapt to what it is hearing. I didn't really expect that. I had envisioned a "jump" with this mapping, but the process is evidently a continuum with my brain calling the shots. So far so good, brain. Keep it up!

Our next stop was a meeting at the League for the Hard of Hearing on 23rd Street in New York. This was the first time I had been to the League since I was hooked up to my speech processor. I am active with the League's advocacy committee, Advocates for Better Communication (*a.b.c.*), but the League has also been my resource for all the services related to my hearing loss for the past 27 years. I was originally referred there by an audiologist/hearing aid dealer when he gave up on trying to fit me for a hearing aid. He couldn't figure out how to fit my fluctuating hearing loss, and he thought that the League would be able to serve my needs better. I also suspect that I was not proving to be one of his more profitable clients.

The League worked with me for about two years, trying to fit me for my first hearing aid. The major stumbling block was my fluctuating hearing loss — a hearing aid that was good one week would be no good the next. I also had what is called recruitment. I perceived sounds as overly loud and uncomfortable, even at volumes that would not bother a person with normal hearing. The result was that what sounded fine in the confines of a soundproof booth was uncomfortable in a normal environment and totally intolerable in the noisy world outside. We finally did settle on something, but for the entire time I was wearing hearing aids, we were always looking for the "right" one. Even my last hearing aid, which I wore for several years, was always considered "temporary" until we could find "it." I ran out of hearing first.

I caught the tail end of the *a.b.c.* meeting at the League, staying long enough to discover that I could function without using the infrared system provided, and rarely even looking up at the realtime captioning, which was also available. I was using my auxiliary mic with my new mappings that I hadn't gotten accustomed to yet. I was shocked, really and truly and happily shocked. Since I wasn't relying on the infrared, it didn't make any difference if people were speaking into the microphones on the table or not, and since I didn't have to stay glued to the captioning screen, I could watch the faces of the people there. Frankly, I hadn't even given any thought to how I would do at this meeting. I knew I was coming in late and I wouldn't be able to "prepare" as has been my custom, finding the best seat to see the captions and the rest of the people at the same time. Between the sound I was getting with my CI, and lipreading, I was actually following the meeting. I think everyone there was as delighted as I was.

After the meeting, I had a chance to speak with a lot of people and, still using my auxiliary mic in this noisy environment, I had no problem doing so. I had been there three weeks earlier, after my surgery but before hookup, and the difference was dramatic beyond belief. Yesterday, I didn't have to struggle to hear. And what better place to have this wonderful experience right after my two-week mapping! The League, and its wonderful people, had always been there for me through my entire descent into deafness, helping me to function along the way. For 27 years, as I lost my hearing, they provided me with hearing aids, assistive devices, lipreading classes, moral support, and most recently, the CI Support Group. At last, after so many years, we had found "it" — the device that was finally able to help me.

My daughter commented, "So that's what you do — come in here, make everyone happy and leave?" Well, yes — but this day was a very long time in coming.

DAY 17
DECEMBER 17

When I got my new map on Monday, I was wondering if it would make any difference in how I would function. Some things are the same, some things are different. I am doing a little better hearing voices at a bit more of a distance — more than three feet away — and I really don't know if it is because of the mapping or because my brain is just continuing to adapt to what I am hearing. For this mapping, we were in a different room than last time, and my audiologist was about a foot further away from me. I'm not sure if this affected the map, but I'm pretty sure it did. The sound from someone further away had a "bubbly" effect and we were able to eliminate that sound quality.

I noticed that some, not all, of the speech sounds on my computer are worse, and I was a little upset about that, but then I noticed that I could hear the television better. Yesterday, I was catching a lot of the dialogue on "Seinfeld" and I realized that the captioning not only omitted words, but entire sentences too! I had always known that the captioning wasn't always exact, but I never realized how much they left out. I noticed there was also some nuance in the tone and delivery of the dialogue that was definitely lacking in "Read Only — Can't Hear" mode.

A trip to the mall last night was easier than the last time I was there. I had written a week ago that I didn't know where to set the speech processor or when to use the auxiliary microphone, and that I was totally bewildered. Yesterday, I knew that in that sort of noisy environment, the auxiliary mic would work pretty well. And it did. The background noise was still discernible, but speech was not drowned out. I'm starting to get the "feel" of what to do although I realize that the sound around me continues to change daily.

I made several phone calls yesterday, and they all went well. I was calling people I had never spoken to before and who didn't know me, and I also spoke to family members. I had the feeling that I was doing a little better than a few days ago. No doubt my confidence is starting to build. When I put in those calls yesterday, I still wasn't sure if I would be able to hear everything, but each successful experience makes the next call easier.

I'm going to have to start some sort of routine of calling friends and family members. Because of my difficulty in using the phone for so many years, and then the cumbersome process of Relay, I have really been out of the loop. Routine communication that would normally occur between hearing people, both friends and relatives, had been effectively put out of my life. I know that hearing people just pick up the phone, say a few words to touch base, then move on with their day. The phone is routine, not a big deal. With Relay, it *is* a big deal. The calls take so long, the hearing person has to speak slowly, they are often asked to repeat and spell — sigh. Relay was a life-saver and kept me functioning and for that I am eternally grateful. But now, I see that I'd like to pick up the phone just to say, "Hi," whether it's to my son, my daughter, my sister or friends. I also watch people move around with their cellular phones and I wonder what they can possibly have to talk about all day long. Just keeping connected, I guess, more of that "not important" conversation. I'll have to try that now — which means, of course, that there is a cellular phone in my future!

I also wrote last week that I was having trouble positioning the phone receiver in the best location over my CI microphone on the head piece. I have figured out that if I hold the receiver, not in the middle, but at the end that has the sound coming out, I have no trouble with this. People had suggested putting a foam ring on the receiver to make targeting the microphone easier, but I find that just holding the receiver at the end seems to do the trick. I have been using my voice mail to test how I'm hearing and what settings on my speech processor are the best each day. I have one message saved in the voice mail just for this purpose.

We went out to dinner with friends over the weekend. My auxiliary microphone is helping me do much better in restaurant noise. From my experience with hearing loss, I know to request the quietest table, usually in a corner. And I know to position myself with my back against the wall, making for an optimum hearing and acoustical environment under limiting circumstances. I was definitely less frenzied than last week. Using my auxiliary mic, I placed it on the table, moving it towards one speaker or another — still experimenting to see what works best.

Saying good-bye to these friends brought up another funny adaptation of dealing with hearing loss that I had developed. When we brushed cheeks, giving "air kisses" good-bye, I had learned over the years always to offer my left cheek. People usually offer their right cheeks, but I always wore a hearing aid in my right ear. When you come that close to a hearing aid, especially a powerful one, it squeals. This is feedback, the same way putting a microphone near a loudspeaker creates that hooting feedback sound in larger sound systems. Whenever I kissed people good-bye on my hearing aid side, I would create this squealing sound, which was embarrassing for everyone. People wouldn't know what to say; I would always have to explain what had happened. It was something I just didn't want to deal with anymore, so I became a "left-cheek kisser." That solved the problem. Now, back to kissing my friends good-bye — I automatically offered my left cheek, and then all of a sudden a lightbulb went off in my head! I don't have to be a "left-cheek kisser" anymore. CI's don't have feedback. I can now be an ambidextrous (or whatever) cheek kisser. A switch kisser!

I was so happy with that revelation, I kissed them good-bye on both cheeks!

DAY 18
DECEMBER 18

I made my second visit to the supermarket yesterday, but this time during the crowded, busy 5 p.m. rush hour. When I entered, I couldn't believe what a noisy place this was, especially compared to the relative quiet of the parking lot. This time it wasn't just the squeaky shopping cart wheels, or snatches of conversation that greeted me — the entire place was alive with noise. Music was being broadcast from speakers everywhere, the entire cash register area was beeping away. I couldn't even distinguish whatever else I heard.

As I made my way through the aisles, I caught snippets of conversations. But my biggest surprise was when I stopped in an aisle to read some product labels. I was engrossed in the fat content of competing brands of potato bread when I heard a faint but clear "Excuse me, please." I HEARD IT, looked up and saw someone trying to get through. I moved over and she passed by my cart, an apparent non-event. But it was far from that for me, someone who hasn't heard those words in many years.

For someone who can't hear, this simple "non-event" is nothing of the sort. I've encountered this situation many times in the past, with varying outcomes. Most people would repeat "Excuse me" louder when their first effort was ignored. It was when this louder call was also ignored that the situation would start to heat up. Some people intelligently realized that their message was not being heard and they would tap my shoulder. Others would become indignant and agitated and try to physically pass, usually muttering something or other, none of which I ever heard. Invariably, I would get stares or quizzical looks like, "What's wrong with *her?*" Having blocked supermarket aisles for a number of years, I think I've encountered just about every type of "passer." Although I had resolved long ago not to let it bother me and to just get on with my shopping, I still always felt compelled to look over my shoulder and keep alert, just in case. So that little "excuse me" that I heard, a non-event to a hearing person, became a non-event for me as well. I just stepped aside. So simple.

With that happy thought, that I would no longer have to worry about blocking supermarket aisles, I wheeled my cart to the checkout line. Instantly I became aware of another phenomenon I had never known about. On my last trip to the supermarket, I was so happy to hear the beeps of the checkout scanner, but that was during a time when there was only one line open. At this busy 5 p.m. checkout time, *all* the scanners were beeping! Was this what everyone routinely hears in the supermarket, a cacophony of beeps? I almost laughed out loud. I never knew this was going on! And since my CI head mic is behind my ear, I was hearing the scanner behind me louder than the one scanning my own groceries, plus all the other beeps in the distance. I guess the cashiers are attuned to their own register's beeps, like mother penguins locating their offspring.

When I mentioned this beeping checkout experience to my daughter, she looked at me as if I had just landed on this planet. And in fact, I had. I had never been to this Land of the Beeping Supermarkets, where one can hear the natives say, "Excuse me, please."

DAY 19
DECEMBER 19

I had my first airplane trip yesterday. With my CI, the experience was a bit different than with my hearing aid. In my communications with Advanced Bionics, the manufacturer of my CI, they recommended that I ask at the security gate to be "patted down," rather than go through the security gate since I might set off the alarms. They assured me, though, that the components of the CI would not be damaged if I went through the gates. Taking their advice, I went directly to the security guard and informed him that I had a "medical device" and preferred to be "patted down." He asked me if I had a pacemaker and I told him it was sort of like that but for hearing. A woman security guard made me stand with my arms out from my sides as she lightly tapped around my body. It took less than a minute. Since I was traveling with my husband, I made sure that he retrieved my handbag from the conveyer belt while this was going on. Once in the airport, I was aware of announcements coming over the loudspeakers, but I couldn't understand them. The announcement to board our airplane at our gate came in a little better since it was coming from speakers directly over my head. I was able to catch a few words, but I would not have felt confident relying on my hearing if I was traveling alone. I would still have had to use my hard of hearing coping strategies.

On board the airplane, the roar of the pressurized cabin was definitely noisy, but not uncomfortably so. With my hearing aid, that noise would have been intolerable. I was used to flipping off my hearing aid and riding in silence, also literally turning a deaf ear to whining children and screaming infants. Now with my CI, I decided to leave it on and use it as a good exercise for "listening in noise." I was able to converse with my husband sitting next to me (even though he wasn't on my better side), but I still had to lipread. I could hear the announcements, but I couldn't understand them. I couldn't really hear the flight attendant in the aisle, but I didn't bother to try because my husband was fielding the questions for me. No sense troubling myself over drink choices in an airplane — not worth the effort. I did hear the chatter of children, but I didn't feel compelled to shut them off. By the end of the flight, I had either gotten used to the cabin noise, or had become numb from it, I'm not sure which, but I didn't notice it the same way I had in the beginning of the flight.

When we got to our place in Florida, I called my children by phone. My husband wanted to listen in too so he told me to try the "speaker" feature, something I had never used before. And, wow — I could hear with that too! So we shared a conversation with our children. I even used "Speed Dial" for the first time.

One thing I did notice was that I had set my CI controls in the morning, and throughout these different listening environments — noisy, quiet, phone — I left the CI at that setting the entire day. This was very different from my experience in the first week after hookup when I had to keep adjusting the volume and sensitivity settings just to stay comfortable. Evidently, it wasn't just a matter of learning how to set the controls, it was also important to get more hearing experience. It was taking time and patience, just what I had been told to expect.

I related in a previous report the problems of feedback with my hearing aid. I forgot to mention that once I had lost my high frequency hearing, I could no longer hear that feedback. If my earmold (the part that fits in the ear canal) for my hearing aid was not securely tucked all the way into my ear, my hearing aid would produce this high-pitched squeal and I wouldn't even know it.

With my CI, there is no earmold so there is no chance of feedback, and I'm certainly not sorry about that! Aside from the feedback, earmolds had always been troublesome for me. The audiologists always thought that a snug fit was best. Unfortunately, snug new molds always produced a suction sensation in my ear canal, which was too annoying to tolerate.

With whittling and wear, I was able to tame the little beasts to fit comfortably in my ear, but it was always a lengthier process than I expected or wanted to put up with. I was even allergic to one of those new improved "Gummi Bear" substances that was supposed to solve all those earmold problems. No wonder I was never eager to get new earmolds!

After many years of use, my last earmold had started to resemble its name and had turned a brownish color that could only come from repeated "waxing." Despite being whittled down repeatedly, it continued to irritate one small spot on the folds of my outer ear. In spite of all this, I still preferred it to the process of breaking in a new mold, so I stuck with it.

Now that I am no longer wearing an earmold, the irritation on my outer ear has finally begun to heal. Not having to deal with earmolds is an added little bonus that I hadn't even thought about before.

DAY 20
DECEMBER 20

I made my first Relay call today as the hearing party! I had always wondered what goes on between the Relay operator and the hearing person during a Relay call. I was calling one of my friends who is a TTY user, so I dialed into Relay, not knowing what to expect. I was worried that I wouldn't be able to hear well enough since the line would be shared by two people (the Relay operator and the person I was calling) and the reception might not be clear enough. I was able to hear the Relay operator and I gave her the number to dial. The other party answered, "Hello, go ahead" and we were connected!

From my experience using Relay, I knew that whatever I said was going to be typed and that Relay operators often complained that the hearing person was speaking too fast. Knowing this, I spoke at a slower than normal pace and this Relay operator had no trouble keeping up. She did ask me to spell the name of a street and she also verified the meeting times I was saying, "10 o'clock to 1 o'clock." This made sense because conveying incorrect information could be disastrous. I got a brief glimpse of what others had gone through for me for so many years of interacting with Relay operators. I could better understand my sister's delight at not having to use Relay with me any longer. She was relieved not to have to stick to vocabulary she knew could be spelled easily, enabling her finally to talk freely about my nephew's Bar Mitzvah.

The hearing party in a Relay call is constrained not only by slowed speech and spelled-out words (or not using them altogether), their train of thought is occasionally lost in the process as well. On the other hand, Relay calling does have certain advantages for the deaf party. I could ramble on and on at full speed, using a cornucopia of vocabulary which could be both expressive and effective. I had the additional advantage of being able to do this without being interrupted until I chose, finally ending my monologues and relinquishing my turn with those two powerful words — "Go ahead."

Using a regular voice phone, will I miss having this kind of control? Not for a second.

DAY 22
DECEMBER 22

I heard music on the radio yesterday, and it really sounded like music. It wasn't quite by chance since it took a lot of fiddling with the radio dials to get it to sound "right." I was listening on a car radio that had adjustments for rock music (bass boosted), jazz (bass and treble boosted) or classical (nothing boosted).

A classical station, with flutes playing, sounded sort of like music, but nothing I'd want to listen to for long. I switched to a jazz station, and I thought that it really had possibilities. I tried all the "tone" controls on the radio, and the jazz setting sounded best. I then tried setting the "sensitivity" control on my speech processor down a bit, and that was better, but putting the volume up on it distorted things. Turning up the volume on the radio was better. After all this experimentation, it finally sounded like music! First there was a guitar playing with a drum rhythm background, and then there was a Herbie Mann flute number. And I really heard it as music! I'm sure it wasn't what a person with normal hearing would have heard, but I wasn't getting a strange electronic approximation. It really sounded pleasant! Thinking about it, we had effectively eliminated the middle frequency ranges, and that seemed to make a difference in the clarity of the sound for me — at least for now.

I guess I'll have to find some Herbie Mann CD's and give that a try. Oh my — does that mean that I can actually go into Tower Records (which no longer sells many records, by the way) and look through the racks of CD's just like everyone else? Stay tuned.

A trip to a flea market brought some unexpected hearing surprises, too. I was purchasing a tray, and after I had given the merchant my money and was starting to walk away, I heard her say, "Thank you. Enjoy it!" "Enjoy it?" Those words really caught me by surprise. I always figured that people were telling me "thank you," but these few added words conveyed a warmth and friendliness that I would have missed if I hadn't heard it. Even lipreading wouldn't have helped me there because I wasn't expecting her to say anything more, so I wasn't watching her face.

I made two more purchases at the flea market, and both times the merchants said something extra that I wasn't expecting. Again I heard, "Thank you. Enjoy it," and "Thank you very much." I had never heard those little pleasantries before, the little words that are like smiles on a face. And it is the little things that do make life a little more pleasant. In this case, to know that someone wasn't only interested in taking my money, but was also hoping I would enjoy the purchase, how nice to hear that!

Now that I've admitted to being a flea market enthusiast, I should own up to being an antique buff as well. Ira and I fell into this interest by accident, and it, too, was directly related to my hearing loss. We could never go to the movies! We had to figure out something to do to take the place of this national pastime. Going to antique shows became the substitute since it didn't seem to require any hearing. It probably would have been cheaper over the years to have gone to the movies, but definitely not as interesting as our quest for antiques and collectibles has been.

I don't feel ready to go to a movie yet, but I can never resist the lure of an antique show. We went to one the other day, and again my CI opened up expanded communication that I hadn't anticipated. I never bothered to talk with the antique dealers before because I knew that understanding their answers would be a struggle at best, but more likely, I wouldn't be able to understand them at all. At this antique show, with my CI, I found myself chatting with a dealer in antique postcards. I started asking her if she had any postcards with a Girl Scout theme, and then we got into a discussion about linen-finish postcards. I started feeling comfortable and happy with this whole exchange, *and then I asked her a question I didn't know the answer to!* I would never have done this before my CI because I knew I would never have understood the answer. I now know that postcards

with a linen finish date from the 1940's and 1950's. But of greater impor-
tance, I now know that I will be able to ask even more questions of more
antique dealers and other people, too! I really feel as if that wall of isolation
has started to come down — that wall of silence — and I am connecting
with people in a way that is still taking me by surprise.

I think I should explain in a little more detail that concept of not
asking a question which I didn't already know the answer to. At the risk of
giving away "trade secrets," I'll explain the fine art of functioning with a
hearing loss in social situations that I had developed over the years. As my
hearing had declined, I had to rely more and more on lipreading. Lipreading
is much easier to do if you know the topic being discussed, so whenever I was
engaged in any sort of conversation, I would try to take the lead and set the
conversation topic. I would also take command of the conversation in the
beginning, asking simple questions, to get used to the voice and speech
movements of the person I was talking to. Then, I would try to ask only questions that either required a simple answer that I could almost anticipate, or
one that it didn't matter what the answer was. I know this may sound manip-
ulative, but over the years, this was the system I had developed and refined,
and — most important — it worked for me.

I can't say I regret having acquired and developed this "fine art of
conversation without hearing." It seems that now I am never at a loss for
words (others might describe it as "motor-mouth"), a trait I probably
wouldn't have had if I had been able to hear for the last 27 years.

People I am meeting now are saying that I look more relaxed and
it must be because I am hearing so much better now. I am finding I have to
tell them that, before, I wasn't hearing them at all, that I was lipreading them
almost completely. I don't think people realized just how little hearing I had.
I was at a party right *before* my CI hookup, and some people thought I had
already gotten my speech processor. They weren't aware of how hard I was
working just to converse with them. But carefully controlling a conversation in a social setting so that it doesn't look controlled, and having to
lipread with almost no sound, is exhausting, both emotionally and physically.
Is it any wonder that I look more relaxed now?

DAY 23
DECEMBER 23

For all the progress I've been reporting, there are still plenty of times when I can't understand what is being said. This often happens on the run when there is no chance to change settings on my speech processor to "tune into" the speech I'm trying to hear. There are also many situations that no matter how much "tuning" I do, I still can't understand.

Some of the people I couldn't hear:

The clerk at a mall Food Court who was reciting salad dressing choices. (The only type I could understand was vinaigrette, so I said okay to that. Less hearing does teach one not to be a fussy eater.)

Someone in a restaurant asking me from behind if I recommended the turkey chile I was eating. (Ira fielded that one for me.)

The clerk in an ice cream store asking me to choose between a waffle cone or a sugar cone. (Ira fielded that one, too.)

From these experiences, I guess I have difficulty either in noisy environments or near food! I mention these negative experiences because I don't want to create the false impression that I am understanding everything coming my way.

Just going about my normal routine still brings unexpected surprises. I bought a magazine, and as I was looking down to put my change away, I heard, "Do you want a bag for that?" My first reaction was, "Who said that?" My brain is not accustomed to hearing things unexpectedly without help from my eyes. At least not yet! I looked up and told the cashier behind the counter that I didn't need a bag for my magazine, thank you. In my hearing aid days, this encounter would have been another one of those tense situations. Since I wasn't looking, I probably wouldn't even have known the cashier was speaking to me, so when I looked up, I would have seen that quizzical look I had seen so often before, wondering why I wasn't responding. Then I would have had to ask if he had said something and then I would have had to try and figure out what it was he said — an awful lot of fuss and stress over a bag for a magazine. Those little stresses seem so insignificant but they forced me to be constantly alert, and really wore me down. But, thankfully, the CI is starting to eliminate those situations.

I'm also noticing that I am turning when people start to speak to me, and with the visual assist at the beginning of a sentence, I don't have to ask people to repeat as much. Someone casually asked me for the time, and I just found myself answering right away — no repeat, no problems. With my hearing aid, this never would have happened. Even if I realized someone was speaking to me, by the time I turned to look, it would be too late to lipread the beginning of what they had said. I would then have to ask for a repeat — at least once, possibly more. Again, an awful lot of stress and fuss just to tell someone "2:45."

I'm still discovering new sounds. When a cereal spoon hits my teeth, it sort of clunks. Both flossing and brushing my teeth have sounds. Who knew that? And I actually had to relearn some sounds. Ira asked me if I could hear the birds and geese outside our bedroom window, and I asked, "You don't have the radio on?" We opened the window, and I really heard them, but they sounded just the way the radio used to sound with my hearing aids — squawks! With my CI, the radio now sounds like speech (not like birds and geese), some of which I can understand, and some of which I can't. And with my CI, birds and geese sound like — well, birds and geese!

We were heading back home, so that meant an airport again. This time I could pick out a few words from the broadcast announcements — not enough to get the message, though. And this time, in the plane, I could hear some of what the stewardess was announcing. I understood when she came around asking for drink choices. I'm not sure if this improvement is because of the voice of the speaker, the volume, the position of the microphone or my brain adapting to the CI. All I know is that I didn't do worse!

After so many years of declining hearing, even to think that I will be constantly improving is still a bit beyond my comprehension. I'm still in awe that I got through the CI evaluation, surgery, hook-up, and can now use the phone and listen to some music. I really can't believe this is happening to me.

DAY 26
DECEMBER 26

They had told me — everyone with a CI, plus the "experts" — that my hearing with the CI would continue to improve for 3–6 months to a year, and even beyond that. Intellectually, I could understand this — emotionally, not at all. My hearing at this point is so much better than it has been for years, I'll guess we turned back the clock at least 15 years. I really can't fathom the idea of it actually getting better than this, yet that is just what is happening!

I made another visit to the supermarket, and going back there at weekly intervals gives me a chance to see how my hearing is changing over time. Now, I know for sure that music can come through those speakers in the ceiling — but not only music, or paging, or announcements either. I was standing in exactly the same spot as I had been two weeks ago, hearing the same sort of beat-like sound — (thup-thup-thup-thup-THIP-thup — thup-thup-thup-THIP-THIP). But now I heard a male voice informing me of the merits of Maxwell House coffee. They beam commercials at you in the supermarket! I wanted to run and tell everyone near me that there was a commercial coming over the loudspeaker! But of course, they all knew, and had known, and had tuned it all out long ago. I'll probably tune it out, too, eventually. But right now, hearing and understanding something that I couldn't hear just a little while ago *with* my CI makes me believe that my noisy world will continue to come into focus.

We were in Atlantic City over the holidays, and I feel like a little kid with a new toy — so many new sounds there, especially those slot machines! I was also delighted to learn that the elevators talked. Remember how surprised I was to learn that they "dinged"? Well, you can imagine my reaction to hear them talking! This one announced the floors, and "going up" or "going down." I know this helps people who are blind, but I couldn't help feeling that if the hotel and casino owners were really so concerned about people with disabilities and complying with the Americans with Disabilities Act (ADA), why weren't there other accommodations, like TTY pay phones in the lobby? These phones are also required by the ADA, but they are rarely provided, in spite of the law. There were amplified pay phones and pay phones at wheelchair height. I'm so happy not to have to rely on TTY phones anymore, but I don't think I'll ever stop advocating for them. I know all too well how it feels to be cut off from the world if you can't just pick up a phone.

And that's the first thing I did in my hotel room, pick up the phone. I was by myself when the phone rang. Instead of that frustrated "What do I do now?" feeling I would have had, I answered the phone. It was one of the friends we were there with, and we made arrangements to meet downstairs. This is my new life, being part of the world I live in, not being left stranded, cut off, alone and dependent.

Answering the phone was just the beginning. We were there with friends and family I had not seen since I got my CI three weeks ago. I spoke with Sam, my brother-in-law, and I actually heard his voice for the first time. I could never really understand him because I couldn't hear his voice and he was very difficult for me to lipread. He kept saying, "You're talking to me!" — and listening and hearing. He's a computer expert, and he knows and understands the complexities of computers and software. But of my CI, he says, "It's a miracle."

I spoke with my sister, Beth, in person for the first time with my CI. She didn't know how to begin. For years she had spoken slower, clearer, louder — whatever it would take to try and get through to me. She couldn't believe all she had to do now was just talk.

I spoke with my friend, Rita, whose voice had always eluded me, and I had found her very difficult to lipread. I used to have to ask other people to tell me what she was saying. Now with my CI, I heard her fine, didn't even ask her to repeat, and it left me astounded that being able to hear her could be so easy. Communication between us had always been such an embarrassing struggle, for both of us.

This was the first hotel I had stayed in since getting my CI, and I didn't have to bother requesting TTY phone service. I knew that now I'd be able to call our friends and relatives in the hotel easily, just by dialing their room numbers. I'd be able to retrieve my voice mail messages too!

When I came back to my room, I saw that the red "message" light on the telephone was on. I guess I must be conditioned because seeing that innocuous little red light made my stomach turn and brought back a flood of memories — all bad. A message left on hotel voice mail could be anything, from an emergency to a hang-up call. There was no way to know until you'd retrieved it. When I had to rely on TTY phones, it wasn't a simple matter to retrieve a hotel voice mail message. It wasn't enough to have a TTY in your own room; the front desk or the hotel operator also had to have one to retrieve a voice mail message. Although, under the ADA, hotels are supposed to have a TTY number to call within the hotel, this rarely happens. I've spent much time and effort trying to make sure that this service is provided. Even if a front desk has a TTY, the clerks may not pick up that line or even know how to use it, so trying to retrieve a simple voice mail message can be and has been a major production. I've often found it simpler to go down to the front desk and have someone there retrieve it for me. But this time, I just pressed the "Retrieve Messages" button on the phone, listened, pressed "2" to repeat, just to make sure I got it right (and also to play with my new toy!). "Meet us at 1 o'clock by the escalator," it said. Simple. Connected.

And I discovered yet another telephone toy. This hotel room had two phones, one by the bed and one in the bathroom. (Makes sense, right?) I was standing combing my hair, and the phone rang. I'd never picked up the phone in a bathroom before. It was my friends calling to meet again. "Sure, no problem. And I'm talking to you from the bathroom." Cool.

As delighted as I am with my CI, I'm realizing from the reaction of others that my hearing loss affected not only me, but everyone who came into contact with me. They are now tremendously excited. I kept hearing, "I talked to Arlene on the phone!" "I talked to Arlene on the phone!" And they were also thrilled just to talk — no struggles, no stress, no frustration.

My family and friends hadn't been able to talk to me like that in years, if ever. And now it became clear to me that they wanted to talk to *me* as much as I wanted to hear *them*.

DAY 29
DECEMBER 29

When I first got my CI, some people who already had them told me that I was really lucky to get mine right before the busy holiday season. This was four weeks ago, and with that very weird electronic sound that I was getting the first week or two, I really had my doubts as to how I was going to make it through all the social events coming up. It turns out that the "veterans" were right. This past weekend was a real test — a social gathering of a dozen or so people on Saturday, and then a noisy crowded cocktail party on Sunday. Quite frankly, if I still had only my hearing aid to rely on, these two social events would have amounted to cruel and unusual punishment.

I always think about the worst punishment that can be dished out to the worst prisoners in penal institutions — solitary confinement. And yet, when a person with a profound hearing loss is thrust into a group social situation, that is what they face. It is such a struggle, that unless they are consciously assisted to be included, they end up in their own silent world, a virtual solitary confinement even though surrounded by people. I have been there many times and it is not fun.

Fun. People always ask if I had fun at this party or that party. When you can't hear what is going on, and your biggest triumph is successfully lipreading your way through some conversations, that isn't what I would call fun. Even discussing this topic with other people who have similar hearing, it never is about having fun — it is always about how well you were able to function. "I could lipread almost everyone there." "I didn't have any trouble with anyone except the guy with the mustache." Triumph over adversity is the order of the day — never fun — in those situations. Then why bother to go to a party? Just not to give in, not to withdraw, not to become a non-person, not to give up on your friends or your family.

That's the scene without hearing, at least what had become the norm for me. But no longer, not with my CI! I wasn't lost in my own thoughts waiting to be rescued and clued in to what was being said or what was happening. I was there! Oh, to be sure, I didn't get everything. In the smaller social gathering, I was able to follow a lot. I couldn't understand everyone in a discussion with eight people talking to each other, but I could follow some of them, and that allowed me to discern the topic of conversation. I could hear enough to be able to lipread enough not to have to withdraw into my own little world. I was most definitely *not* in solitary confinement.

I also noticed how often people were tapping me — touching me — to get my attention. I really had them well trained, and they were so wonderful not to forget! But I'm still wondering why I'm noticing it now when it seemed so routine before. I think it has something to do with that solitary confinement I spoke of. That tap on the shoulder, or touch on the elbow was the lifeline that brought me out of my world of silence. It was a welcome tap, a welcome touch that said that someone cared enough to include me in what was going on. But now, I remained connected by sound, by hearing speech — even incomplete speech — and I wasn't dropping out. If I hadn't dropped out, I didn't need to be brought back, so those touches now seemed unnecessary. It's similar to ringing the doorbell after someone's already opened the door.

I'm wondering what to do about all the folks that are conditioned to get my attention this way. When they tap me and repeat things for me now, I'm finding myself telling them I heard them the first time. This happened at the social gathering this weekend, and then also in the car, listening in on a cellular phone conversation between my husband and my son and also listening to a conversation with others in the back seat. When they asked me why I didn't indicate that I heard what was going on, I really didn't have an answer. I didn't know how to react myself. I hadn't expected to hear it either! I'm also not used to responding; I had gotten used to being in my own silent world. But I'm starting to come out. And I figure the more

I start responding, the less people will tap and touch. It will all gradually fade away. Not to worry, this "problem" will take care of itself.

The crowded noisy cocktail party was actually the answer to my dreams and expectations. I had been asked before getting my CI, "What are you hoping for?" I wasn't asking for much. All I really wanted to do was be able to get enough sound so that I could lipread easily. Bingo! Wish granted at the cocktail party yesterday!

This party was very noisy, lots of people and music in a room filled to capacity. I was using my auxiliary mic with the sensitivity set low and the volume set at a comfortable level. I clipped the auxiliary mic onto my jacket about half-way between my waist and chin. If it's too near my mouth, I sound too loud to myself which makes me speak too softly. I wanted to try to leave the auxiliary mic on my jacket rather than hold it because a) I'd have two hands free to eat and drink with, and b) it really is more elegant looking. I figured that I would give up on a drink and elegance if I needed to hold the microphone closer to people's mouths, but I thought I'd give elegance a chance first. And, no problem! I would say that I was hearing from 40-50%, depending on the person, and lipreading the rest. This probably doesn't seem too successful to a hearing person, but I had become accustomed to lipreading 90-95%. With 40-50% sound, I can lipread with little difficulty. This noisy party was a "worst case hearing scenario," too, with plenty of leeway for more hearing by moving the auxiliary mic if need be. So this was a huge success. People who have known me for years said that my face looked so much more relaxed. I'm sure this is true. I don't think anyone ever realized exactly how I was functioning before, how my brain was working on overdrive — lipreading, controlling conversation, figuring out what was going on — just to make casual small talk.

"So, did you have fun at this party?" I never did before, and I'm not sure I did this time either. I was wondering too much how I was going to do. But it was pleasant, that I will say. I was able to chat fluidly with most of the people there. I knew not to stand next to the musicians — it doesn't take a genius to figure that out. And it was mostly one-on-one, actually an easier listening situation than the smaller social gathering of the previous day.

A word about elegance. It is becoming apparent that with this waist-level speech processor, certain types of clothing "work" better than others,

especially if I'm going to be wearing the auxiliary mic for noisy environments. Garments with buttons down the front are best for clipping on the
auxiliary mic. I really wanted to wear a chic black fitted jacket to the
party yesterday. I hadn't worn it since getting my CI, and when I first
tried it on, I looked pretty lumpy. But I really didn't want to give up on this
jacket because — well, because. So I fiddled with placing the speech
processor at various locations on the waistband. Putting it all the way to the
side made me look absolutely W-I-D-E. So I put it right in the front, but that
made me feel like a mama kangaroo. I inched it over a bit — to about
"10:30" — and voila! That was good — still a little lumpy, but it didn't pro-
trude in front or side silhouettes. And with the auxiliary mic clipped
inconspicuously between two buttons, I was all set. I know people will say
that it's the hearing that counts, not the cosmetics. Absolutely correct. But
why not go for both if you can?

DAY 31
DECEMBER 31

As December comes to a close, it has been exactly one month since I received my CI speech processor. I hadn't anticipated sharing this experience with so many people, but I have received many comments asking me to please continue writing. Just yesterday, several people responded to my comment that partying with a profound hearing loss was tantamount to cruel and unusual punishment, saying that it struck "a strong chord" and was "punishment as usual." Nancy K. wrote, "Sad to say, this type of scenario is 'cruel and USUAL punishment.' I'm glad you're one who finally escaped!" And Rachel F., who was having her CI surgery the next day, wrote that "all of a sudden, the faintest glimmer, the smallest light comes on and the possibility presents itself that maybe just maybe, it won't have to be like that for me forever!" So I continue.

The other day I heard the microwave oven beeping from two rooms away. I'm finding that I'm hearing other things that are out of my range of sight. I heard the television in the next room, a conversation from another room, even the faint sound of the television downstairs. Some of the sounds have me perplexed because I'm not sure what I am hearing since I can't see their source. I'm still a bit dubious that I'm supposed to be hearing all these things, and again wonder if medical science hasn't gone overboard with its bionics. At any rate, the fact that I can hear more than I could a few days ago means that the "experts" are right again, and that my hearing continues to improve. I had thought that meant simply in clarity. The idea of having a greater range of hearing, while leaving the volume levels set on the speech processor, is something I hadn't anticipated.

The UPS driver came to my house to pick up a parcel and I responded to the doorbell with no problem — that's an old trick. I was able to understand the driver fine as he was speaking to me, and even when he looked down to fill out a shipping form. He kept asking me questions and I kept answering him, even though I couldn't see his face! My brain was on alert again — "Hey, where is the visual information? You're supposed to see his face!" I have always had to tell people to please look at me when they spoke so I could read their lips. This had become so routine that, standing there answering questions without looking, all I thought of was "when do I get to tell him about my hearing problem?" We finished the transaction, smiled at each other, said thank you and good-bye. As he walked back to his truck, again I thought, "But, I didn't get to tell you I have a hearing problem." I didn't have to.

Again, this may sound trivial to those new to this game, but I have had to tell virtually everyone I came in contact with that I had a hearing loss, and how best to communicate with me. This included people that I had never met before, even people that I would know for only a few moments. So, not to have to do this anymore, I realized that I had gotten my privacy back. You, Mr. UPS Driver, do not have to know anything about me to deliver your package. Of course, you may have missed out on my advice about assistive devices that your father or grandmother with a hearing loss might have needed. But right now, my life is my own and it just became a little bit easier.

With these new hearing experiences, I trekked back to the supermarket (yes, the weekly supermarket report!). I wondered what new things I would be hearing this time, considering my new improved bionic range. When I entered, it didn't sound all that loud to me, even though it was very busy there. I instinctively wondered if my hearing had diminished since the last time I was there. No, the cashier area was beeping away, there was music coming over the loudspeakers, the shopping cart wheels were squawking, children were giggling, and I could hear snatches of conversations. Someone even asked me where the cranberry sauce was. I guess he got my attention by voice. I had to ask him to repeat, but got it on the second try when I was looking at him. So, I was still hearing everything. I must be getting used to it all.

DAY 33
JANUARY 2

Sound is beginning to change some more. This morning there is a f-f-f-f-f sound coming out of my speech processor. I can lessen it by turning down the sensitivity setting. I doubt anything changed in the speech processor overnight, so it must be me. I wonder if it is related to this widening of my hearing range. The sensitivity affects range, so if I have more of my own, the settings on my speech processor are probably not accurate for me any longer. My telephone ring and the modem hookup sounds have changed as well. Before, I just heard those sounds as one unified roar; now I'm able to discern a variety of individual tones that weren't there before. The modem hookup is a high and low electronic symphony — so much going on just to get connected! The phone ring is also a melodic blend of electronic impulses, and long, too. Is it possible that I didn't hear the whole ring before?

A new experience entered my life, shopping for CD's! It was the last day of Chanukah and I thought it would be a real treat to take my daughter, Emily, to Tower Records to buy a CD for her, and one for me too! I didn't have to ask her twice — teenagers' most precious possessions are their CD collections, and they would never turn down an opportunity for more. For me, the whole idea was a new adventure. Again, something hearing people take for granted is just not the case with me. There was never any reason for me to be in Tower Records (the mother of all record stores, a misnomer since they sell mostly CD's and tapes.) I had been in there a few times buying gifts, but of course never anything for myself. I actually hated that place. There was nothing in there for me and it was one of the few places that made me feel truly sad. I didn't usually harbor any "woe is me" feelings during my long descent into deafness. While it would have been nice not having to put up with declining hearing, I always did what I had to do and didn't dwell on what might have been. Except in Tower Records.

It wasn't only that I couldn't hear the music, it was also that I had no chance of being able to hear the music. No captioning, scripts, studying or trying harder would ever make me hear those CD's. And it was also the culture of the place. Here was a whole part of our culture that I was excluded from. I think that's what bothered me. There was no making up for hearing when it came to listening to CD's or the ritual of buying them. It was hopeless in there, and that's how I felt too.

It was an excellent idea taking Emily with me for my first CD-buying trip. A seasoned teenager, she knew the ropes, and the locations of what I was looking for. I knew from listening to the car radio that I wanted a Herbie Mann jazz flute CD since the high pitches of the flute seemed to sound pretty much like a flute and the lower accompaniment was pretty much like music too. I wanted to start with a sure thing, not to set myself up for disappointment.

The store was crowded with teenagers and vacationing college students, and I thought I would feel out of place. I don't even have pierced ears, much less pierced eyebrows, nose or navel. But as I watched all these young people trying to appear very New Age, I was smug in the knowledge that although they might be trying to look like the future generation, I was BIONIC. Now that has to be the cool of cool!

Emily picked out some rock masterpiece that we later tried in my car's CD player. I actually caught some of the lyrics! In addition to my jazz flute selection, I also bought Prokofiev's *Peter and the Wolf* because it has both spoken dialogue and several different instruments playing individually, an arrangement that's easier for me to hear. I listened to it right away in the car, and the winds and percussion seemed to be coming in sort of like music, but the strings (Peter's theme) were just noise, nothing musical about them at all. Time will have to tell on that.

New Year's Eve was a listening pleasure. At a dining room table for six, I was doing fine. Even though I couldn't understand without looking,

I could easily understand anyone I paid attention to. Evidently, a certain amount of hearing is needed to be able to understand a conversation without being told the topic being discussed. Having that degree of hearing now means that I no longer feel isolated or go off into my own little silent world. This makes a huge difference in how I feel and how I view social interactions. I am actually looking forward to socializing more, even thinking about planning activities that include *people*. And I'm looking forward to calling them up to make these plans.

I thought this subtle changeover would happen, especially with the phone. I have been calling a few friends, opening the avenues of communication. I know that, before, I had been reluctant to place calls by Relay, and I'm sure other people had felt the same way. With this reluctance, communication slowed down or stopped entirely.

How to explain what I'm feeling? I want to talk to people. Yes, I want to. I think it is natural. I'm reminded of what Helen Keller said about her deafness, "It is an inhuman silence." She was right. I was there, but now I'm back.

DAY 34
JANUARY 3

We rented a video movie yesterday, as is our custom. They are closed captioned, so I can read the dialogue on my television at home. I haven't ventured into a movie theater yet, and I haven't been to one in years because the local movie houses don't show captioned movies (not yet anyway).* This was the first time back in the video store since getting my CI. I'm discovering that no one lets you shop in peace anymore! Piped-in music — this store had it, and so did the drug store next door. I guess the marketing experts must know something I don't about sensory stimulation and sales.

The video store has never been an easy place for me. Picking out the videos is not too difficult if you can remember what was considered a decent movie months ago when they were first shown in the theaters. It takes that long for the video version, complete with captions, to appear in stores. The problem with this shop was that the cash register didn't display the amount of the sale, so the clerks had to tell you how much you owed. I never understood the amount said even when they weren't looking down at the computer when they were talking. I had given up on hearing them long ago and resorted to the "change" strategy of purchases. By giving the cashier a $10 bill for video rentals, it didn't matter how much it actually cost. (I knew it wouldn't be over $10.) Of course, I couldn't check if I got the right change that way, but it was worth it.

This time, with two videos in hand, I thought I heard the cashier say, "Six ninety-seven." I wasn't really sure, but on principle, I didn't want

*Since this was written, several local movie theaters have started showing captioned films.

to ask her to repeat. So I used my "change" strategy again just to make sure. I watched her open the drawer, put in my ten, and remove one, two, three singles, and then one, two, three pennies. Yes!!

The movie we watched was "Michael" with John Travolta in the starring role as an angel, with feathers and all. I was able to follow the dialogue with the captions on my tv screen, and I could even hear the music! Music was a big part of this movie and although it didn't sound as wonderful as it should have, it was still recognizable as music. I could even "get" the musical joke of playing the "Chicken Song" whenever Michael, the angel, was dancing, with feathered wings concealed beneath his coat. I really would have missed a lot of the detail in this movie without the music. That triggered a remembrance of having been there and done that before — missing the music.

Last year, I took out "Mr. Holland's Opus," a movie everyone was raving about. I was especially interested in it because it is about a high school music teacher, and both my parents were high school music teachers. The storyline was fascinating and the acting was wonderful, but I couldn't hear the music. The music was very important to this movie, and I wasn't able to hear it. That would have been upsetting enough, but one of the featured songs in this movie was "Someone To Watch Over Me." That's the song that Ira and I danced to at our wedding, and I couldn't hear it anymore. For over 27 years Ira had watched over me as my hearing went from normal to deaf. I was consumed with sadness as we watched that movie, not because of the movie's story, but because of our own story. I think it's time to take out "Mr. Holland's Opus" again, and listen to it.

DAY 35
JANUARY 4

Another day, another story. I thought this would let up by now, but life is actually getting more intriguing the more I use my bionic ear. We were invited to a party at a friend's house, people that we have known a long time. We hadn't seen them since I got my CI, so they were very anxious to have us come.

I knew the party would be a noisy situation, so I hooked up the auxiliary mic at home, clipping it inconspicuously between two buttons on my cardigan sweater, which I was wearing over slacks. So except for the tiny little auxiliary mic sticking out, I looked "clean." The funny thing is, though, that with the CI cord going down my back and out of the way, I feel liberated and don't even think about the apparatus on my head. All I have is the concealed speech processor at my waist, which in this day and age of beepers, everyone seems to have anyway.

When we got to the party, our friends were anxious to see my CI, where it was, what it looked like, and most of all, if I could hear them. Of course, I had just taken great pains to look "invisible," so they were surprised not to see much of anything other than the tiny auxiliary mic. They were really happy that I could hear them, since trying to communicate with me had become so difficult.

What I noticed at this party, which I hadn't expected, was that no one else knew about my hearing history or my recent CI experience. I was just another person to be introduced to. I made conversation with a variety of people, not even asking for repeats. Totally fluent conversation.

"Heh, heh," my brain started talking to me again. "They don't know you're really deaf. How would they know? You are conversing like a hearing person, you look like a hearing person, you're not talking about hearing, and you even sound like a hearing person. Ergo — you are functioning as a hearing person!"

That part about not talking about hearing is the crux of the matter. If you have to tell people that you need to see their face to talk to them, or that your hearing is very poor, or any such declarations, then not only are you condemned to your hearing loss, you are also sentenced to talking about hearing forever. It's inescapable! After you've finished explaining your own situation and they marvel at your guts and lipreading ability, they invariably have a great-aunt, grandfather, or mother-in-law who needs a hearing aid or an amplified phone or plays the television too loud. And since you know all about that stuff, that's what you end up talking about — all the time. (Talking to people about my CI, when they are interested in finding out about it, is different. That's a pleasure!)

So at the party, I didn't mention a word about hearing. I didn't talk about my CI; I didn't talk about the miracles of modern medicine. I talked about the town we lived in, curly hair, Florida real estate, exercise routines — all the drivel that people talk about when they don't have to talk about hearing. I was really enjoying myself too, as if I had finally made my escape. Then I found myself in a four-way conversation in the living room.

One fellow was leading the conversation and rambling on about golf. (You would too if you had an 11 handicap.) I was following the conversation, participating in the discourse, laughing appropriately, and not asking for a single thing to be repeated. I don't think I got it all, but all wasn't necessary; I was doing great. Then this fellow started to tell a funny story, which began to take on ethnic overtones. He seemed a little uncomfortable talking out loud about the "politically incorrect" vocabulary he was using, so he stopped and asked, "Can you read lips?"

You mean he had no clue that for the past 27 years I had been enrolled in the Lipreading School of Hard Knocks and had just graduated? That if this party had been just five weeks ago, I would have been struggling to lipread him and we would probably be talking about hearing instead of golf?

So I replied, "Sure, I can read lips. Go ahead!"

With that reply, I felt like Eliza Doolittle in *My Fair Lady*. No one suspected her past, and not only did they think she was a "lady," they thought she was a Hungarian Princess. And that's exactly how I felt, but not only a Hungarian Princess, a Hearing Hungarian Princess!

I could only think of what Dr. Hoffman had told me in the hospital after the surgery when I felt so awful from the anesthesia. He said, "But you're going to hear soon!"

So — Congratulations, Dr. Hoffman* and the Cochlear Implant Team at New York University Medical Center. You did it! You did it! You said that you would DO IT, and INDEED YOU DID!

---

*Dr. Ronald Hoffman is now Director of Otology, and Medical Director of the Cochlear Implant Center and Balance Disorder Center, Beth Israel Medical Center, New York.

DAY 36
JANUARY 5

I went to visit my mother today. She lives almost two hours away, a drive that I used to find very difficult. If you can't listen to the radio or to tapes or CD's, there is nothing to do other than steer a car in silence. I would always have to stop and buy myself a caffeine soda to keep alert. This time, I was actually looking forward to the ride. It would give me a chance to listen to my two new CD's, *Peter and the Wolf* and Herbie Mann on jazz flute.

As always, I was curious to see if anything had changed in my hearing since the last time I listened in the car. I could follow *Peter and the Wolf's* narration pretty well, missing some words here and there. I especially noticed consonants I hadn't heard clearly in years. "The big grey wolf came out of the fore-S-T." The British narrator said "forest" so distinctly! Now that I mention it, I am hearing myself say those sounds more distinctly too. My speech had always been good, but I wonder if it will be a little more precise now that I can monitor those sounds.

The flute, bassoon, percussion, and oboe sounded fine, pretty much as they should. The volumes varied — the flute sounding the loudest, so things are still far from settled. I had difficulty with the clarinet volume particularly, barely hearing it at all. What did surprise me was the string ensemble for Peter's theme. Last week I reported that it sounded like electronic wind. Now it was recognizable as music, and I could follow the melodic line. I can't say it sounded like strings, but it was in there somewhere, surrounded by electronic noise. Maybe next week or the week after, the string sounds will emerge.

I have been noticing that after listening to music for a while, my hearing tends to fade out, no matter how I fiddle with the volume controls. On this particular trip, I noticed this on the return trip home. I guess the nerve just says "enough is enough." This had been happening on the telephone too, after about 10 -15 minutes, but now I find I can talk (and listen) for over half an hour without this "fade-out" phenomenon. At this point, I can only observe and make notes, to get an idea if this is something which will eventually work its way out, or something I will have to work around.

I finally reached my destination, and although I still can't declare myself an enthusiastic long-distance driver, at least I wasn't bored to tears. My mother, who has Alzheimer's disease, lives in an assisted living facility, which accommodates her needs. When I greet her, I no longer wait to see if she's going to recognize me, so I always say, "Hi Mom, it's your daughter Arlene." This orients her, and on this visit, she greeted me with a big smile, hug and kiss. "Oh, Arlene, how good to see you! How are you feeling?"

My mother has always asked me, "How are you feeling?" She first started doing this when I got married and left home, which was also when I started to lose my hearing. She has never specifically asked about my hearing, but only how I am feeling. I'm not sure, even now, whether these were code words because she didn't want to bring up the subject of hearing, or whether she was simply concerned about my general health. On this visit, she was true to form and asked how I was feeling. Without a second's hesitation, I replied "Good!" She did a doubletake and so did I. In over 25 years of her asking this question, I had never answered "Good," only "Okay." I would really mean "Okay — but," with the "but" being my declining hearing. I was coping, managing, and that was okay, but it was never good as long as I continued to lose hearing. My hearing loss had truly cast a pall over my life. With the boost my CI was giving me, I really did feel good.

My mother would always introduce me to her friends, but I was never able to hear them. Meeting these people was not something I looked forward to; it was awkward and I felt I didn't want to work so hard for trite pleasantries. In these situations, my mother frequently functioned as my interpreter since I always understood her voice, no matter how bad my hearing got. That would have worked out okay, except that with her short-term memory being so poor, if I didn't get her to repeat something immediately, she would forget what was said and then get flustered and upset. This reminds me of my grandmother's philosophy. When she was asked, at an advanced age, how she was feeling, she would reply, "There's so much wrong, you have to laugh!" And that was just the situation I faced having an Alzheimer's patient for an interpreter.

My intuition about feeling good with my new-found hearing was confirmed when my mother introduced me to a lovely gentleman, the maintenance man, who described himself as the "master of the miscellaneous." Without any assistance, I heard him tell me what a lovely mother I had, and though she may not remember things, she was a wonderful person. He also mentioned writing a poem about her, which he said he left in her room.

No wonder I was starting to feel "good." On a routine visit, instead of walking in fear that someone would talk to me and that I wouldn't be able to understand them, I was given a gift of love and compassion that made accepting my mother's decline just a little bit easier.

DAY 37
JANUARY 6

I had my fourth mapping today, five weeks after hookup. My speech processor holds three programs, yet during the past three weeks, I had settled on the one which functioned best for me.

At the mapping session, we went through the routine of setting my threshold and maximum comfort levels, and then my audiologist tried a program which was essentially the same as the program I had preferred before, but with the expanded settings. I'm starting to get the hang of this now, and I'm realizing that stronger and more powerful is not necessarily better. I know now that when I'm asked to find a comfortable volume, it should really be comfortable, and not the loudest that I can comfortably tolerate. If the resulting program does happen to be stronger and more powerful, it is only better if it fits my particular auditory needs.

I told my audiologist that speech was starting to take on a "husky" quality, and she adjusted something to make it more natural-sounding. We had the option of keeping my old favorite program or trying two more. She tried another program with the high frequencies boosted, which sometimes helps people to understand speech better. And the third program was the same as the first but with no noise suppression.

We tested all three programs by repeating sentences without looking. It was really remarkable. As well as I had done last time, repeating the sentences this time was much easier. I didn't seem to have to think as hard to hear the words, and didn't feel that I was getting any of them from context or guessing, so things must really be improving.

We then tried the favorite program I had come in with, but that didn't seem to have the depth of sound the new programs did. So throwing caution to the winds, I chucked the old tried and true, venturing out with the new software. As she loaded the new programs into the speech processor, we chatted — no sound, all lipreading — and for the very first time, I felt that I wanted my sound back. I needed my sound! My world is now a world of sound.

Once out in the real world, I started to have second thoughts about dropping the old "tried and true" program. Everything was louder, bigger. From inside my car, I could hear a truck's engine revving, not just an anonymous roar. The radio news didn't seem as clear, or the music either. But then I reminded myself of my "fade" problem, especially after intense listening situations, so maybe my nerve was just tired. Or maybe my brain needs time to adapt to these new settings. I'll have to give it all a chance. I also filed away this information for next time; maybe making things less "husky" made the radio less clear.

The program without the noise suppression seems to work better for music. But the jury is still out on these mappings, and I will certainly know more by my next appointment, in a month.

Armed with a whole month's CI experience, and a little hesitancy over my new mapping, I attended a meeting, my first full meeting with my CI. There were about 15 people there, and real-time captioning was provided, but no assistive listening system. I was really curious about how I would do; I had no idea what to expect. As soon as the meeting began, I knew right away. I could follow what was going on. Oh, I still had to look at who was speaking, so I still had to lipread, but I think that I missed very little. I glanced at the captioning to check myself on several occasions. What I found interesting was that I fielded the chairperson's voice from about 10 feet away. The whole sense of the sound I was getting was far different from a hearing aid's sound. This CI had range, something no hearing aid I ever had possessed. I didn't have to fiddle with volume controls to pull in that sound either. It was just there waiting for me to hear.

DAY 38
JANUARY 7

Three things on my Wednesday agenda: haircut, telephone conference call (!), and a Broadway show. The big challenge was the telephone conference call, but first things first.

The CI is useful almost everywhere, but it can't get wet or damp, so a simple activity like getting a haircut commits one to silence once again. I'm used to this because it's the same way with hearing aids. The switch from CI to silence, though, is far more dramatic. From a full range of sound, I'm plunged into silence, a much bigger change than removing an essentially ineffective hearing aid.

I have been going to this beauty parlor for years, primarily because it is a friendly and accommodating place. The owner himself has a hearing loss, and the warm tone he sets in his shop makes me feel comfortable there. I am used to lipreading my hairdresser, even upside down when getting my hair washed, and she is always patient and understanding. Contrast this with another beauty shop owner that I had dealt with, who wanted me to make my appointments in person so she wouldn't have to deal with my Relay calls. I wasn't her customer for very long!

My CI presents a few changes in my routine. First, my haircut still has to camouflage the patch of hair that was shaved for the surgery. The other consideration is that the microphone/magnet headpiece shouldn't get wet, so I have to make sure that my hair is dry before putting it back in place. That's not a big deal; it just takes a little longer. Having encountered no problems at the beauty salon, I got ready for my next adventure, a telephone conference call. How in the world was I ever going to deal with that!

I knew that I could now hear most voices on the phone, but this was going to be a four-way call. I'm a member of the New Jersey Arts Access Task Force which is part of the New Jersey State Council on the Arts. I represent the New Jersey Division of the Deaf and Hard of Hearing Advisory Council on this forum, and I've been drafted to serve on the planning committee of an upcoming Arts Access Conference. As a member of a four-person sub-committee, it was decided to try a teleconference rather than have everyone drive a distance for a very short meeting. I agreed to try it. Why not!?

The preliminaries were sent via fax. The appointed time was 2:00 p.m., and I was ready. The phone rang right on schedule. It was an AT&T operator setting up the call. She gave me the phone number to dial and the conference call code numbers, just in case I got cut off. This was so amazing! Numbers, which had always been the most difficult for me to hear, now come in easier than words. While I was taking down all this information, with no repeats, I kept wondering how I was doing this, getting information orally only, using no visual cues. I was flying, but I was wondering what was keeping me up!

Then I waited, and two female voices came on the line. This was starting to get more difficult but I was still in there swinging! I knew both of the women from in-person meetings, but I had no clue as to which voice belonged to which person. I had never heard them before! The lone male voice completed the group's attendees on the line. We decided to start with the concerns I had raised first because I told them I wasn't sure if my auditory nerve would start to "fade" on me. While I was involved in the conversation, I could follow it. When the other three people were talking between themselves, I could only get words here and there, but still had an idea of what was being discussed. Not bad for a first-ever!

I would do this again, if necessary. It worked well enough for me to be included in this type of communication. The other members of the committee said they were giving me a crash course in telephone use. They certainly did, and I survived.

Completing the agenda for the day was the Broadway show *Titanic*, shown with open captions and with an infrared listening system available in the theater. I had tried using infrared systems twice before, but without success. The sound had been either too loud or too soft, never quite right. On a friend's suggestion, I got a different patch cord, the wire which connects my speech processor to the infrared receiver.

I was all set, with appropriate cords plugged into appropriate sockets, and awaited the start of the overture. I knew I could still enjoy the show with the captions, even if the infrared didn't work for me — so I was essentially doing triple flips with a safety net. Bless those captions!

The lights dimmed and the overture began. Ira looked at my face and one glance told him all he needed to know. My eyes were wide with wonder and my mouth first dropped open and then turned into a broad grin. "I can hear it with the infrared, and it sounds like music!" Now, I'm not sure if what I was hearing would have qualified as music to everyone. All I can tell you is that it was not electronic wind and I didn't want to shut it off.

The dialogue was difficult to understand because it was mostly sung, so I followed the captions for most of the show. Sometimes I understood it, but checked with the captions anyway. I later learned that a lot of hearing people had trouble understanding the lyrics and relied on the captions as well. It seems all my forty- and fifty-something friends are pleased to accompany me to captioned shows. They won't admit to needing the infrared and are not up to hearing aids yet, so captioning is a pretty subtle and elegant solution.

As I think about my Broadway debut with infrared, the technology that made this possible is absolutely mind-boggling. Start with the actors on the stage, who were wearing cordless body mics. Whatever they were singing or saying was beamed to the theater's sound system. The infrared transmitter was also plugged into this system, and it turned the sound into invisible infrared light which was beamed out into the audience. My infrared receiver picked up the light signal, converted it back to sound and fed that into my speech processor, which converted it into impulses which set off the electrodes in my cochlea which stimulated my auditory nerve which made my brain hear the actors on stage — instantly! I think Rube Goldberg would have been impressed. And with all these technological marvels happening in that theater, the *Titanic* still sank — again.

DAY 46
JANUARY 15

We're in Florida, taking a respite from the winter up north. One of our favorite activities is exploring the state park system here, a wonderful collection of preserves that bill themselves as "the real Florida." Their purpose is to preserve the natural flora and fauna that existed here long before condominiums, shopping malls and M-I-C-K-E-Y obliterated most of it. We visited MacArthur State Park which is just north of Palm Beach, right on the ocean.

We picked this park because it had a picnic area, nature trails, a visitor center, and boardwalks to the ocean and beach. Like everything else with my hearing loss, we had always gravitated to activities like nature walks and picnics because no hearing was required to enjoy them. You don't need hearing to stop and smell the flowers or read about them in a self-guided nature trail. You also don't need hearing to pick out an idyllic spot to peacefully munch on delectables.

This park had a lovely secluded picnic area. I enjoy the peacefulness that comes with getting away from humanity. We chose a table completely surrounded by big palm trees and palm fronds, and spread out our goodies. Long ago, we had developed the tradition that no picnic is complete without potato chips, and the Pringles variety have become our picnic staple. As we sat there in our private jungle, I knew this picnic was different right away.

There was a constant breeze blowing — of course, because we were near the ocean. But it rustled the leaves of the trees, a musical accompaniment in our private dining "room." Then there was a bigger rustling sound, almost a roar. "What's that, Ira — an airplane, a truck?" No, it was still the wind, but a larger gust, rippling the treetops near us. I have been pretty good at identifying sounds, but this one mystified me; how could the wind be so loud, as we sat in what I thought would be quiet seclusion.

My quiet was interrupted once again as I started to eat my Pringles. CRUNCH — crunch, crunch, crunch. Potato chips! Of course, they crunch! Along with the sensory delight of this traditional picnic food, there was now a sound to enhance the experience. I had asked my daughter if I'm supposed to be hearing myself chew and she told me, sure. I don't recall ever hearing myself chew, so this sound must have been so ingrained that I never realized I had lost it.

Picnic finished, we made our way over to the nature trail and a boardwalk which took us through a mangrove forest, then up over the dunes to the beach and the ocean. There were no concession stands or commercialism in evidence. The beach was nature as it should be — unspoiled. Along with the ocean vista that I was familiar with was the sound of it now, the constant rush of the waves lapping the shore. And there was the wind, the whoosh of the wind. I made sure it didn't hit my microphone directly, which would have created that harsh sound that microphones without foam wind-protectors are prone to. As we walked along the beach, it was as if the sound track had been added to my silent movie.

When we went back over the dune into the mangrove forest, it suddenly became quiet again. Could that be right — so quiet? Ira said, yes, it was very quiet now. I had to check, so I retraced my steps and went back over the dune out towards the beach. LOUD again. The idea of sound added to our nature walk was intriguing. Nature walks had always been quiet.

As we walked back through the mangrove forest, I heard the gentle rustle of the leaves overhead, like the tinkling of tinsel. A curious thought crossed my mind. I had always gone on nature walks because I could enjoy them without any sound. Now that I was aware of just how much sound there was, I wondered if someone without sight could enjoy the same walk, just listening to the ocean waves and breezes.

My thoughts turned to a beautiful Hebrew song and prayer that I first heard in my temple fourteen years ago, when they had just installed an infrared system there. I could hear the music so clearly then, and the words. It was sung first in Hebrew and then in English — *Eli, Eli.* It was special then. It is even more special now.

> O Lord, my God,
> I pray that these things never end:
> The sand and the sea,
> The rush of the waters,
> The crash of the heavens,
> The prayer of the heart.
> The sand and the sea,
> The rush of the waters,
> The crash of the heavens,
> The prayer of the heart.

DAY 47
JANUARY 16

We've gone to the movies once already, and it wasn't a disaster, so we thought we'd try another one. My attitude towards going to the movies seems to have changed dramatically. I'm optimistic now, and whatever I'm missing, I can hope to try and get next time. After all, things are improving and every opportunity to practice in various listening environments could help my brain to adapt some more. This is a far cry from the mind-set I had while losing my hearing. Then, no matter what I was hearing, I could only look forward to *less*. Movies were not only frustrating to watch, they were also harsh reminders that worse was yet to come.

We wanted to see *Titanic*, the movie, and this time we were prepared. We found a movie theater that was supposed to have an assistive listening system. We agreed that if the system wasn't working, or if I wasn't understanding enough to enjoy the movie, we would leave. The theater had an FM system with receivers that I could easily plug my CI into. We took the headphones and decided that Ira would try them out first to see if they worked in the theater. The concession stand had already checked that the batteries were charged and that it was "on" and set to the correct channel. We took a seat on the left side so that my CI microphone was closest to a speaker, just in case the FM system didn't work.

The movie started, and — nothing, nada, nil. Ira said the FM headset wasn't working, so it was futile for me to even try it. I had heard so many people complain about these assistive listening systems not working. Now I knew their frustration. I should have informed the management, but the movie was starting, and I didn't want to miss the beginning. I was also curious how much, or little, I could understand without an assistive device. This movie was three and a half hours long, so if I was not understanding enough, it was going to be torture.

I can't say I did great. There was a lot of background music, and I just couldn't field the words through the music. I did get some of the details, and even hearing the music gave dimension to the story line. The string quartet, playing on the deck of the sinking *Titanic*, sounded like a string quartet. Perhaps also because it looked like a string quartet. Just a guess here, that by *seeing* strings, my brain is more inclined to *hear* strings. I must be getting fussy because everything is sounding a little too tinny for my taste. Can yesterday's miracles seem ordinary so fast?

I didn't give up in despair, even though I was missing a lot of dialogue. I was catching enough to wonder what I would catch next. Unlike my hearing aid days, I wasn't discouraged. This movie was a good one to see at this stage of my hearing odyssey. It is largely visual and I would even recommend it to deaf and hard of hearing people who don't usually venture into movie theaters. There are details in the story that would be missed without the dialogue, but it's not really crucial. The ship sinks anyway.

We had now experienced the *Titanic* sinking on the Broadway stage and in the movies. From a purely artistic standpoint, it was interesting to be able to compare the two, noting the way movies can replicate the reality of the disaster, yet live theater can involve you on a more personal level.

This was my second try at a movie with my CI and maybe one day I will actually find a working assistive listening system. For all the money ($200 million!) that was spent by the movie studio, and the technology involved, ensuring that the *Titanic* would sink realistically, it would be nice if they could get a simple FM system to work in the movie theaters.

On a positive note, I'm starting to know the movie-going ropes a bit — the way to buy a ticket, head for the popcorn stand, find the correct screening room, and pick a good seat. I did learn one more thing this time. After sitting for three and a half hours with no intermission, I could barely move. My knees were stiff and other parts of me ached. Ah, the benefits of going to a regular movie theater instead of renting an outdated video!

DAY 48
JANUARY 17

Back at the airport; let's see what comes through this time. Announcements in the corridors are still a blur. Getting "patted down" is now routine. I heard a new sound, a beeping noise which I had never heard before. Little did I know it was coming from an airport tram, something like a golf cart, that they use to transport people through the hallways. It nearly ran me over before Ira yanked me out of the way. So much for hearing sounds from behind! That's a quick lesson right there — it's not enough to be able to hear it, you also have to know what it is! I'm wise to this beeping now and ready for it next time!

Sitting at my gate, I heard the overhead loudspeaker announcing an adjacent flight. I couldn't catch much, just a few phrases, something about volunteers and final boarding. My goal is to be able to hear announcements so I can travel on my own without asking for assistance. I must be getting a little closer because I heard my own flight's boarding announcements — not all of it, but enough to know which seat numbers were boarding, and the flight number, and "LaGuardia." This is progress. But I'm also getting the hang of this. Just by being able to tell that the announcement is coming from the overhead speaker at my gate, I know to look at the gate clerk who is making the announcement. That would enable me to lipread the announcement if I had to.

On the plane, I heard much of the flight attendant's spiel about the life vests and such, and an announcement about the closed overhead bins being full and the open ones still having room. And I heard the captain talking about Charlotte, S.C., and Chesapeake Bay, and Washington, D.C. and Wilmington, Delaware, and New Jersey, and LaGuardia. And then I heard that it was 37 degrees, and that we were landing at Gate 3, and which carousel the luggage would be at.

I'm mentioning all the specifics because when you ask anyone on an airplane what the flight attendant or the captain is saying, they always tell you "nothing important." There is nothing more important to a person who can't hear than what he is not hearing! So to all those people who have never heard these announcements on an airplane, this is what they are saying. You decide if it is important or not. There seems to be a progression here. If you can't hear it, it's very important. If you've never heard it before, and you're hearing it for the first few times, it's important. After you've heard it many, many times, it becomes unimportant and you start to wonder why anyone would want to know what they are saying.

Not to give a false impression of success, I didn't catch some of the announcements at all. Slow and steady, I guess, is how we would describe this process. I can't say I'm disappointed, or even frustrated, when I can't make out what they're saying. Even though it is still hit and miss, I'm starting to get used to the hits — happy too, but still wondering if today's miss will be tomorrow's hit. No crystal ball here, just another reminder that it will take more time and more patience.

DAY 50
JANUARY 19

I'm starting to get a feel for which situations are easy for me and which give me trouble. When I listen to the radio, some reports don't come in at all, yet some come in very well. Hit and miss again. I'm also still amazed that numbers are so easy to hear, easier than other words. The weather report, or the stock market report, are easier to understand than the news or talk programs.

The funniest turn of events is that hearing in the car — without looking, so it can even be dark — has become one of my easier situations, perhaps because I've been in vehicles that have pretty quiet interiors. This is a dramatic departure from what I had become accustomed to with my hearing aid, where I was virtually non-functional in a car. I would always have to look at who was talking, but turning around to the back seat was not only inconvenient, it was usually not worth the trouble since it was always iffy whether I could lipread whoever was back there anyway. And forget about the dark. That was a lost cause altogether.

Now, I make sure that if there is a choice, I position myself in the front passenger seat. My head mic is on the left side of my head, so that makes it easier to understand the driver, which so far has been my husband. Since the head mic faces the rear, I can hear most passengers in the back seat, without looking, even at night. Absolutely amazing!

The strangest scenario has been to listen to the conversation, hear a question, and then answer it. What's strange about that? I was never able to do it before and it absolutely floors Ira, who is still used to me sitting there in bored silence, especially at night. I have to admit, he has stopped jabbing me so much to get my attention. I figure that this behavior will work its way out sooner or later. The more I answer to my name, the less I get jabbed.

What I didn't expect was actually hearing my name. One would assume this would be a routine sort of experience, but the truth of the matter is that not only had I stopped responding to my name as my hearing declined, but people actually stopped using it. Why would anyone bother to call my name if they knew it wasn't going to do any good?

What is happening now is that people are starting to use my name instead of tapping and jabbing me. I am learning what it sounds like to hear my name, and it is not only Arlene. Sometimes I'm called Arl, or Arlie, depending on the situation or who is doing the calling. Who ever thought I would remark about appreciating the fact that there is now a purpose to having a spoken name!

The most difficult hearing environment by far has been noisy restaurants. I've been in a few recently and I'm never quite sure how to deal with it. I know that my own hearing is changing, and what may work one day doesn't work the next and each restaurant presents slightly different variations on this listening challenge.

There are certain rules that carried over from my hearing aid days and number one was to find the quietest part of the restaurant, taking a seat that wasn't surrounded by people talking. The goal was to have as little background noise as possible. Rule number two was to use the auxiliary microphone with my CI, which I had also used in my hearing aid days. The microphone picks up what it is close to, so is effective in blocking out background noise when I turn down the sensitivity setting.

Now, the fun begins — trying to hear the other people at the table. I really don't function well in this environment, and my lipreading skills are put to the test once again. To be sure, I field much more sound than I ever did with my hearing aids, even when they were working for me, which in the past year or so, they were not. I find, too, that I've changed my standards — a lot. I used to consider it a success with my hearing aid if I used my auxiliary mic one-on-one with a person, putting it close to their mouth, or clipped to their lapel. I can say with certainty that I would now be able to hear very well if I wanted to use the mic in that way. But I'm not really willing to do that anymore. I just don't want to. I really want to be able to converse with people on both sides of me, and also across the table. Boy, do I set tough standards! Well, if we are going for miracles, then let's go for them! The time is still early and I figure, let me try to train my brain and (I was going to say ears, but they are sort of bystanders here) nerves to understand in this environment. Maybe it's not so great today, but I'm hoping that I will tilt the balance more and more each time — more sound, less lipreading. I think that is an obtainable goal, and at seven weeks after hookup, I still have the enthusiasm to go for it.

DAY 51
JANUARY 20

This was a very full day, with a lot of "firsts" with my CI. Thinking about the succession of small events that make up a day, it is incredible how hearing figures into just about every one of them, and what a difference it makes not to have to struggle with each one. There is also some turmoil going on between my brain and this speech processor. It has been two weeks since my last mapping, and my brain has decided that it doesn't like two of the programs very much anymore, the ones that have noise suppression on them. Although I can hear on the phone with these programs, the sound coming in is too muffled compared to the program that doesn't have noise suppression on it. But everything has also started to sound too tinny and has taken on a raspy quality, no matter which program I choose.

The problem with using the noise suppressionless program is that I have to turn the sensitivity down to eliminate some of the background noise, and that changes the balance of how I am hearing. I'm trying to explain this but the reality is that I don't know. I'll talk with my audiologist tomorrow and see what she suggests; either live with it or move up my next mapping appointment, which is in two weeks.

Okay, let's run through the day. I figure that I'll use the louder program. I hear sounds that I can't identify, but I can try moving closer to the source. I'm in the bedroom, walking to the wall, getting closer to the sound. It takes me to the hot air heating vent. I'm hearing the heating vent blowing hot air, and I know that it is near the furnace, so I think I'm hearing the furnace also. Who needs this? I turn the sensitivity down a little. The furnace disappears. Good.

Getting into my car for the first time in almost two weeks (we were away), I immediately flip on the radio to see if my CD's sound any different. My heart sinks — the CD's sound awful, and I had hoped they'd be better! I fiddle with the programs and the controls, but nothing seems to help. What is this? Herbie Mann isn't playing his flute and the accompaniment is garbage. Peter and the Wolf are a mess. I shouldn't have left them alone together!

I flip to the news station. Okay, that's still coming in clearly. I stay tuned to my old favorite, CBS News Radio 88, and sit and listen for a while, experimenting with the settings. I can understand the news, so I didn't lose that. I can't believe that the music has left altogether, so I bravely tap the CD/Tape button again. And, lo and behold, Herbie is back playing his flute! It's a little raspier than I recall, but he's there. And the Wolf and Peter seem to be getting along better now, the way I heard them two weeks ago. Don't ask me to explain what happened. It seems that my brain forgot how to listen to this stereo system and needed a little time for it to kick in again.

Driving into the city, I listen to the radio and the CD player the whole way. They talk very fast on the radio, but I'm able to follow most of it if I concentrate. Before going up to the meeting at the League for the Hard of Hearing, I stop at a luncheonette to buy a sandwich. I have been there before, pre-CI, and it was always difficult to know what they were saying. This time I hear the clerk say "a dollar fifty." I was watching her as she spoke and I doubt that I would have heard her without looking; it was very noisy there. But the point of the matter is that I didn't have to ask her to repeat, and it wasn't a big scene just to buy a bagel with vegetable cream cheese.

I have a meeting with people I hadn't seen since right after my hookup and some whom I hadn't gotten a chance to speak to at all since then. I am noticing that I hear the "s," "d" and "t" sounds much more distinctly and my tongue is making certain to mimic what I am hearing. I'm not consciously doing this. It just seems natural to repeat the sounds the way I hear them. I've noticed that even at night, after I've taken my CI off, I am still making the same effort to form those sounds, even though

I can't hear them (or anything) without my CI. It feels different to me and people are telling me that my speech is different. It wasn't bad before, but it has a different tonality now. And they also tell me that my face looks much more relaxed. Before, I had to strain and use every wile in my head just to figure out what people were saying. Who in the world could relax under those circumstances?

At the meeting, I again function pretty well by listening, watching the speakers, and using the captioning to catch what I missed. After the meeting, with everyone talking to each other, it is very noisy. I feel that rather than struggle, I'll put on the auxiliary mic since that blocks out the background noise so well. I don't like to wear it all the time, and in general situations, I prefer to do without it. If it is clipped onto my clothing — as it is now — and I put my coat on, it doesn't pick up very well. Clipping it onto my coat is cumbersome, and it makes annoying noises rubbing against my clothing. So on my way out, I put it away.

Waiting for the elevator, I enjoy hearing the "ding." I didn't have to frantically scan all the elevators to see if any had arrived, or which one. I always felt like some sort of cat on the prowl doing that. This seems much more civilized. My prey announces itself!

On the way home, I figure I'd hit a lot of rush hour traffic, so I'd stop at my favorite hot dog wagon before leaving the city. You can pull up to the curb, roll down your window and get the food and beverage of your choice. Today, I feel like treating myself, so I ask the vendor for a knish and a soda. I've stopped here many times before and the fellow knows me. He's always said something to me, but I've never heard him. Today, he tells me it's two dollars, and wishes me a nice day, with a smile. Those little pleasantries again, much nicer than bewilderment, or wondering whether you should respond, or if you've given him enough money. Pulling up to a street corner in Manhattan, you don't want to get caught up in long transactions, so short and sweet is best — and safest.

And the ride home is full of news, weather, Herbie Mann, Peter and the Wolf. Still not great music, but at least back the way I had left them.

DAY 53
JANUARY 22

I was at the car dealership because my car key clicker wasn't working right. I asked one of the salesmen what I should do and whom I should see. He gave me detailed instructions — go right over there, down the stairs, through the door, to the left, and speak to Thomas or Don. Normally ("normally" will still mean with a hearing aid until functioning with a CI becomes "normal" for me), I would have stood there and explained my hearing loss, asking to repeat, over and over until I figured out what to do. Not this time. I only asked for verification on the names, Thomas and Don. Any lipreader will tell you that Don is a ridiculously difficult name to understand. Not only is it a name, which could actually be anything, but it is only one syllable, so you can't see much on the lips. I heard it right. I followed all those left-right instructions, actually found Don and resolved my car key clicker problem.

Thinking about that "Don" success, I keep noticing that the consonants — s, d and t — are much clearer. I noticed it while watching television too, and that made a difference in understanding some of the words. Listening to the news seemed to be easier than listening to the dialogue from a regular program, probably because all newscasters face front, with their faces in full view, with no background music.

I spent a lot of time on the phone today. The priority was a call to my audiologist to get an earlier appointment for a remapping. Even though I can still hear on the phone and do well in general, things have changed too much in the past two weeks, and everything sounds far too tinny and raspy, with music starting to sound worse, instead of better. Rather than "toughing it out," I put in a call and got an appointment in a few days. We'll see what happens then.

Speaking about the phone, I made a few calls to people I had always called by Relay. Nice surprise for them! It's hard to explain that even though you can hear on the phone, you are still really deaf! When that speech processor comes off at night, the world is silent — very silent.

A visit to a travel agent I had used months ago was also interesting. I didn't mention my CI, but she was wondering why I was sitting there so relaxed talking to her, not asking for repeats. The last time we spoke, I was hunched over her desk with my auxiliary mic in hand trying to field whatever little sound I could. Nice change.

I'm making this sound too easy, though. The truth of the matter is that I can't really count on the hearing yet. There are too many different hearing situations, and I'm not settled with my mappings, programs, settings or brain yet. So I don't have real confidence in this; there's still too much up in the air. I was told that the first three months are filled with change, so I can't say I didn't expect it. I just don't want to create the impression that you plunk on this device and hear as if you never didn't.

I even have that feeling of uncertainty when making phone calls although, so far, my track record has been fine. I haven't had to bail out of a phone call yet. Some people are easier to hear than others, and some connections are better too. I still ask for repeats, but not all that many. A funny turn of events is that I like all those phone menu options — the press one this, press two that. For some reason, those options come in very well. Maybe it's one computer talking to another, like friends. Even if I don't understand something, there is usually a "press something" to repeat, so I can stay on the line as long as I like. With a hearing aid, and especially through Relay, those phone menus are a real problem. They are all spoken too fast to understand with a hearing aid, and with Relay, the operator can't type the options fast enough, so you usually have to wait for a human, which slows the process down even more. Of course, sometimes you don't get the human option either, so that takes even longer.

I used to make all my Relay calls in one sitting, serial calling. It would take only one call into Relay and I'd stay with the same operator for all the calls. I must have gotten into that habit because I'm still making my calls in one sitting. I finally figured out, genius that I am, that I don't have to hang up the receiver each time I want another dial tone. Why did it take me so long to figure out that I only have to depress the button that the receiver rests on? It's been a while, I guess.

There's a lot more time in the day because the calls take a lot less time! Leaving a message on an answering machine is much quicker. With Relay, you'd have to have the operator type the outgoing message to you, then it would be too late to leave your own message because by that time, the line would disconnect. So the Relay operator would have to dial the number back again, and prompt you when to leave your voice message. It's good that the service was available, but much easier to hear the message, and the beep, and leave a message. I can't even estimate how much less time phone calling is taking me, but it is significant.

The realization of the day is that with my CI, my ears have become totally ornamental! They are vestigial structures now, useful for hanging earrings on and for resting the frames of my glasses.

DAY 54
JANUARY 23

How can every day bring a new hearing adventure?

I had two meetings to go to today, a tight schedule with overlapping times. I figured that I could stay for most of the first one, then head to the second and catch the last hour of that one. My plans were scrambled by the weather; it was sleeting, with the promise of more to come. I'm not really thrilled to drive in bad weather. Nothing is that urgent to risk life and limb.

I bundled up warm, took my furry mittens, brought boots, and got behind the wheel of my car. But this time, I had something at my disposal that I never had before getting my CI — my car's radio. I immediately tuned into the news, the weather report and the road conditions. I wanted to know what to expect later in the day. The weather in my area wasn't all that bad, but driving a distance, that could easily change.

They predicted more rain with sleet, heavy at times, with temperatures in the thirties so it could turn icy too. There were tie-ups on the roads caused by accidents. It wasn't very comforting to hear that they were finally clearing away the tractor-trailer that had jack-knifed somewhere in the New York Metro region. The New Jersey Turnpike was having problems at Exit 14. It was generally a mess out there.

So, based on those reports and looking out the window during my first meeting, I decided to stay put, stay until the end of that meeting and head back home, instead of going still further from home and risking worse driving conditions.

This was the first time in memory that I have used the radio to make a decision like this. Usually, I would have just the morning newspaper or online weather report to go on, no traffic reports and weather updates. Looking out the window was the only way I would have been able to check the weather conditions without my CI.

Because of what I heard, I made my decision. I made an informed decision because I was informed. This is something I never seriously thought about — until today.

I was attending a New Jersey Arts Access Task Force meeting, the first one since getting my CI. The last time was incredibly difficult because I was barely functioning with my hearing aid and I had to use all my wits just to be there. This time, everyone knew about my CI. I was greeted, literally, with open arms. I had teleconferenced with a few of the members but this was the first time I was hearing their voices in person.

I had hooked up my auxiliary mic for the occasion because the room had a bare floor and the acoustics had quite an echo. I could understand a few people's voices very well. If all the voices were like those, that would have been a pleasant surprise. Others were not so easy, so my lipreading skills were needed. I was able to turn to the voices and so could catch what they were saying as they spoke. On a few occasions I asked for verification of what I had missed and to make sure of some information, but I was in there hearing — far from perfect — but far from the mess I had been last time. I was only at a loss when more than one person spoke at a time. I didn't really have a chance with that.

For this group of people, I gave the "short course" in what a CI is and the basics of how it works. I thought that it was important that a committee, whose agenda is accessibility for people with disabilities, should know what a CI was all about. Particularly important was explaining that I could use my speech processor with an infrared or FM system, accommodations which are useful to other people with a hearing loss also. It sounded funny to declare myself "bionic" because we are so used to that term being used in futuristic science fiction. But the reality is that this is no longer science fiction. It is science fact, and I am, in fact, bionic. The future is now.

DAY 56
JANUARY 25

I am starting to get some confidence, knowing that I will be able to hear, for sure, in most circumstances. This gives me the courage to try out my new hearing, risking disappointment but still willing to venture out.

With the weather not too cold over the weekend, we set out for the antique/flea markets on 26th Street in Manhattan. There is always a strange mix of junk and treasure there, and careful combing has produced finds in the past. These markets had always put me in an awkward position. When I had only my hearing aid to rely on, I was hesitant to engage the dealers in any kind of conversation, even to ask to look at something that was locked away. I would ask for price, sometimes, but little more. From my positive recent experiences, I have loosened up a lot, but I still have to consciously tell myself that I can now request to see something, that I can ask about it, and that I may even hear the reply. I am certain now that I will not have that sinking feeling of "what am I going to do now?" that I would get when I couldn't understand the dealer I was speaking with. Because I'm confident that will not happen anymore, my behavior is starting to change. I am coming out of that stifling shell of silence.

I used my new hearing, and courage, to ask one dealer about something I didn't recognize. It was a "perfumer," a purse-sized perfume bottle. I heard her say the word, while I was looking at her, and I got the information — first time, no repeats. Each success paves the way for the next encounter, and that was to find out the price of a 1950's-looking lorgnette — rhinestone-studded folding eyeglasses with a handle. I didn't intend to buy this item, but I was curious to find out how much they wanted for it. That's what I could do now — find out things on a whim. I wasn't sure who the dealer was in this booth, but one of the customers pointed to a young man who had his back turned to me.

Now, this is Manhattan, and some of the dealers, and many of the patrons, do not look like they just came from Kansas. Some look downright strange. And strange is definitely how I would describe this dealer. When he turned around, he was all hair! He had a mangy mane of matted braids sprouting from all parts of his head. They covered his eyes, and most of his face. Where the mane left off, the mustache began, covering lips, teeth and mouth. A full beard completed the visage.

To the uninitiated, this is a lipreader's nightmare; you can't possibly lipread a face full of hair! Thoughts raced through my mind. Should I ask the price of this trivial rhinestone-studded trinket? Was it really worth trying to communicate with this furry head? Sure, why not! So I asked, "How much?" not knowing if I was going to hear the response. There was nothing to lipread. There were no lips.

And then came the words, "Twenty-five dollars." I got it! I really heard this hairy thing say twenty-five dollars! I didn't want it for twenty-five dollars, but I could reject it because I knew how much it cost and not because I had no chance of finding out! That is the difference hearing made, another tiny detail adding color and dimension to my day.

Television is starting to come in a little better now. I'm still following the dialogue with the help of the captions. I am not really much of a television-watcher, remnants of the days when there were not many captioned programs. I pretty much stopped watching television in the mid-1970's when "The Dick Van Dyke Show" and Mary Tyler Moore were in their heyday, with twin beds in the bedroom. I didn't resume until most of the prime-time programming was captioned in the late 1980's. Imagine my shock at finding "Married with Children," with its pseudo-pornographic content. What a change had occurred in my absence!

I never became a channel surfer or a serial program-watcher. I have always preferred to pick out a program, watch it and then leave or turn off the television. Unfortunately, I never had "control of the clicker," and watching someone else surf the channels was not much fun. Annoying as watching snatches of 50 programs was, at least it used to be silent! Now the 50 programs have sound — 50 snatches of irritating sound along with the visual images. I'll have to figure out what to do about this. I'm not sure I want to get used to programs flitting past my eyes AND "ears."

After the regular prime-time line-up of captioned programs, the news came on. The captioning for the news is in real-time, which means that it is captioned as the news is reported, because it is a live broadcast. Real-time captioning has a time-delay since the person doing the captioning has to hear what is being said before transcribing it. I found myself getting frustrated by watching the captions. I could hear some of the newscasters, which was made easier because they are always facing front, but I became impatient that the captions weren't keeping up. I never felt impatient before, but then again, I never heard any of the newscast before. So I think there is a subtle transition going on here. I'm going to be listening to the news, checking what I hear with the captions, but I'll probably start relying more on the sound, and less on the captions. Stay tuned.

As for the news, I hadn't really heard a news broadcast, or bothered to listen to one, in over twenty years. I don't even remember the last time. And look what I get to inaugurate my "news-hearing" with, the Clinton sex/impeachment scandal. They can talk about this on television? Actually say these words — out loud? But then, that's the same sort of jolt that "Married with Children" gave me, which just goes to show that Life probably does imitate Art.

And on to the Super Bowl! I couldn't understand any of the television commentary! None! The entire broadcast had the roar of the crowd in the background, and I couldn't pick out any speech at all. It was just noise. Maybe next year.

DAY 57
JANUARY 26

I had made an appointment a few days ago to be remapped because I sensed that things were out of kilter with my present programs. The programs with noise suppression were not fielding speech for me as well as they had been although I could still use the phone with them. Sounds had become very tinny and raspy. I started using the program that had no noise suppression even though it was not as good in the presence of background noise. I could go on and on about how I kept fiddling with settings and adjusting the best I could, but it was clear that after two weeks, my hearing had changed.

This appointment was three weeks since my last mapping and eight weeks since hookup. The session went as usual, setting the threshold and comfort levels. There had indeed been changes in those settings and we tried to get things to sound less tinny and more natural. I've gotten used to the reality that nothing monumental is going to change with these adjustments. The big change occurred when I first got the speech processor and the rest is a gradual evolution. My range is expanding, but from day to day, map to map, I am resigned to the fact that there is not going to be a sudden surge which will move me dramatically past the difficulties I am still encountering.

That said, I am growing very accustomed to what I can hear and I'm starting to get a little impatient with what I cannot. After eight weeks, is the honeymoon over? Not really, the romance is still there. I love this CI for liberating me from my prison of silence. As my faithful partner, I am coming to depend on it, knowing I can count on it to hear in most situations — sometimes better, sometimes worse — but I am confident enough to know it isn't going to let me down entirely. This is not trivial! There were some activities in my life that I just *didn't do* — period! — because of my hearing. Now, with a sense of confidence that I can hear, I'm starting to make up for lost time.

Take, for example, a simple walk around the block. New neighbors had moved in across the street not too long ago and I had never gone over to welcome them or introduce myself. I had waved from a distance when passing by, but there had never been any verbal exchange. This was not by mere chance; it was by calculated design. I hadn't introduced myself because I didn't want to be put in a position of not hearing the response. Life was stressful enough without looking for new sources.

The walk around the block today was different. No fear! I saw my new neighbor loading her car. I thought twice about stopping to talk, rather than just waving. Should I? Could I? Yes. "Hi, my name is Arlene and I'm your neighbor who lives over there." I heard her say her name was Susan, and it turned out that they had moved in about a year and a half ago. Now we're really neighbors. That gave me a very nice feeling. It must have been nagging at me for a year and a half. The previous neighbors had come and gone after living there four years and I had never known them.

I still love the sound of acorns underfoot, but now, I'm up to people. As I kept walking, I saw another neighbor pull into her driveway. Our children used to play with each other all the time. I could have simply waved and avoided human contact, as I had been doing. But this time I didn't want to. I waited in her driveway until she got out of her car and walked over to me. We hadn't had a face-to-face conversation in years. As we caught up on how our children were doing, she commented that I was hearing her quite well and she immediately realized that something was different. It still surprises me that this hearing business has so much impact on the people that have to communicate with me. Being able to hear makes it much easier for *them!*

I had lunch in the city with two friends, Anne and Emily, alumnae of the lipreading class we attended several years ago at the League for the Hard of Hearing. We had vowed to stay in touch, and have been meeting periodically ever since. Each time, my hearing was worse. I'd have new gadgets to help me cope, but the lunch dates became more and more difficult. I would have to use all my wits to be part of the conversation while they would try their best to keep me connected. There was no escaping the fact, though, that if they said something to each other, I could not follow unless they repeated it for me. It was clear that I was sinking with each encounter.

Our luncheon rendezvous was their chance to see for themselves how well I was doing with my CI. They, too, were doing well with their hearing aids, the new digital variety — computerized. We all knew the strategies of effective coping skills, which presented the dilemma of how to sit three hard of hearing people at a table, all with our backs to the wall! Answer: you can't. But a corner table enabled two of us to sit against a wall, and overall, it was the quietest spot in the room. I used my auxiliary mic and I was doing fine, hearing and lipreading, and following everything. It was such a happy luncheon. I was back. Actually I was better than I had ever been since these two friends had known me.

The successful use of our new electronics was not the only cause for celebration at this luncheon. This was one of those regular activities which were my constant reminders that my hearing was always getting worse. I wonder how conditioned I had become to that fact of life, that 27-year fact of life. When I had contemplated getting the CI, that was one of the considerations: that downward spiral would end at last. I would finally have a level of hearing that I could depend on, whatever that turned out to be.

With this luncheon, I was experiencing the outcome of those expectations. It had taken me eight weeks to get to the point where I could rely on this device, that I could predict pretty well how I was going to hear with it. If everything stays the way it is now, that in itself would be such a dramatic departure from what I had been conditioned to expect. But no, "they" say things will still continue to improve, albeit slowly. I'm not sure how that will happen. I do know, though, that I can look forward to hearing at least as well at the next luncheon with my friends.

DAY 58
JANUARY 27

The news of my CI and my improved hearing is starting to get around. Those not on my email circuit are getting the news the old-fashioned way — by phone, mail or in person. I called my aunt up on the phone and she was happy to hear from me, but then asked, "How come I'm talking to you like this?"

Did you ever wonder what the Indians were thinking when the Pilgrims landed? "Who is this, how did they get here, and from where?" It's not that different, I imagine, receiving a voice phone call from someone who is supposed to be deaf. Can I stretch a metaphor and suggest that it is, indeed, a whole New World?

I had thought that not using Relay would give me more time in the day. As I expected, my "chore" phone calls are taking a fraction of the time that Relay does. What I hadn't expected was that people stay on the phone and chat. Nobody ever really chatted with Relay. Okay, so I don't have all that extra time that I used to spend waiting for Relay transcriptions. It's being replaced by meaningful and sometimes not-so-meaningful human contact. That is something I didn't have before, and it is adding to my essence as a human being.

DAY 59
JANUARY 28

I'm beginning to get the idea of how mappings work. When I left with my three new programs last Monday, they sounded fine in the quiet of the audiologist's office. Initially, I had expected the maps to instantly fix things that I had been having more difficulty with, like music or listening in noise, or just clarity in general. I'm finding that it doesn't really work like that. The mapping process creates new settings which increase the probability that I will do better. Not necessarily instantly, but as my brain adapts to them.

I'm mentioning this because the first thing I have been doing after finishing with my mapping sessions is to get into my car and turn on the radio. The traffic noise and radio always sound different after the mapping, and I can't say that they always sound better.

As the days pass and I start to get used to this new map, little things start to sound better, whether it is something in noise, or something about music. There is a process going on, and it is not a "quick fix" sort of procedure. My gut reaction had been to be disappointed that the "new map" wasn't producing new gains right away. I'm learning not to get disappointed, at least not at first. I am just starting to get wise to this game. All the advice and warnings about time and patience were just words until I actually experienced the very subtle nature of it all. I get the feeling that we are painting a masterpiece here, and one would not want to rush a masterpiece.

A visit to my mother once again was much easier because I could now hear what people were saying. The little things are so important! As my mother and I took a walk through the living areas and corridors of her senior residence, I heard people calling her name. "Hello, Beulah," "Hi, Beulah," and I also heard the comments of people who knew her. "We love her. She's wonderful." I had never heard this before, and she has been living in this facility for a year and a half.

She started to sing as we walked hand in hand down a hallway. She was a high school music teacher so music is her language. I could hear her as we walked along and we could converse easily, even though I wasn't always facing her. She started to ask me about my — and she gestured to my ears and body to indicate whatever it was that I was using now that enabled me to hear. I said it was going wonderfully well.

We passed a door in the hallway with a plaque on it that read, "Bless this house, oh Lord we pray. Keep it safe by night and day." I asked her if she remembered the tune that went to that verse. It was something that I had grown up with because one of the radio programs (WQXR, I think) that my father had always listened to signed off with that prayer. She didn't remember it at first, but then I sang a little for her, and she caught the tune and began singing the whole thing. This was a positive moment. The Alzheimer's progression continues, but being able to reminisce about a melody and a prayer with my mother was a good experience that my newfound hearing enabled us to have together.

DAY 61
JANUARY 30

As I begin to repeat activities, I'm noticing that I can sometimes hear sounds that I couldn't before. But things are still hit and miss. What is a little strange is that sometimes I can hear things coming out of loudspeakers and sometimes I can't. There doesn't seem to be much rhyme or reason to it. We were walking along in a noisy antique show in a convention center, and I heard loud and clear an announcement warning that the cafeteria would be closing in 45 minutes, and the snack bars would remain open until the show closed. Why could I hear that and not the announcements in the airports? Hit and miss! I keep rooting for the hits, hoping for more of them, and fewer and fewer misses.

Dining out is another recurrent activity and I seem to be getting the hang of it, using my auxiliary mic. I had an interesting variation on this theme when I was having lunch with my friend, Joan. Joan has always been very accommodating of my hearing. She was one of the few people ever to ask me, "What can I do to make it easier for us to communicate?" a simple question that literally lifted some of the burden from my shoulders and put it on hers.

The restaurant we were dining in had some background noise, so I was pleased to be functioning fine under these circumstances. Someone Joan knew came over to our table, and they started talking, first to each other, and then to me. Before getting my CI, this would have been one of those "tune-out" situations. With my hearing aid, there was no way that I could lipread two people talking to each other, so it had gotten to the point where

I wouldn't even try. By habit, I started to tune out again. But then I realized that when I was looking at these two people talking to each other, I could follow what they were saying. This hasn't happened to me in years — to share a conversation, unplanned and unassisted, between two other people! And because I could follow what they were saying to each other, I could answer appropriately when the conversation turned to me for introductions and comments. It made me feel like a regular human being. The woman who came by had no idea that this was momentous for me, that it was extraordinary not to need someone tell me separately who this was and what they were talking about. This was typically a situation where I would have needed an "interpreter," and I didn't need one.

I went back to a shopping mall again, this time with my daughter. We were chatting as we parked the car and walked along window shopping. It wasn't until we got to the food court that I realized that I hadn't touched the controls on my CI. I had figured from my previous mall experiences that I would be popping on that auxiliary mic in just about every noisy environment. This time I didn't seem to need to turn the sensitivity down or reach for my auxiliary mic. That was a pleasant revelation, and also a change worth noting.

DAY 63
FEBRUARY 1

I was hooked up with my CI speech processor on December 1st, but I hadn't seen my son in person until yesterday. Michael is 23, and lives on his own in Boston. We had spoken on the phone several times, so he knew how well I was doing. He said he was enjoying talking to me on the phone, without Relay, and it was something he could get used to very fast. It was obvious to both of us right away that we could communicate much better by speaking to each other directly.

Michael had missed most of the beginning bumps in my road of trial and error. When we finally saw each other face to face, it was as if I had never had a hearing problem. He just walked into an "easy listening" environment. I am now fairly comfortable with this CI, and beginning to simply use it and not make a fuss over it. So our family conversations are now much easier, with no special attention as to why. I like it this way — just blend in — no special treatment or accommodations to talk to me. Michael was still conditioned to touch my arm to get my attention. It's a nice thing to do anyway and I have resolved not to "correct" anyone. If they want to touch my arm or wave a hand, that's still all right with me. These conditioned behaviors will work themselves out, just the way they had worked their way in — gradually.

With both my children together in the back seat of the car, I got an unexpected treat. I could hear them talking and I could follow the family conversation. This was the first time ever for me because by the time my children were old enough to hold conversations in the car, my hearing was far too poor to understand them. When I was driving them to their many after-school activities, I never heard them talking to each other. Maybe that was a good thing when they were growing up. I think they will probably tell you that they have some special sibling secrets that are truly secret because they knew that Mommy couldn't hear them. Maybe they bonded in a way they never would have had I been able to eavesdrop. Not everything is terrible about not being able to hear.

My successful use of the phone continues and I have yet to bail out of a phone call. Some connections are better than others and some people are easier to hear than others. Sometimes I have to ask for repeats, but for the most part, there are no significant problems. That is not to say that people sound the way they used to on the phone. I'm still amazed that I am understanding because, frankly, the sound coming in is still rather strange and electronic. I can usually distinguish male and female voices and if I know who is talking, I can imagine what they really sound like. But if I don't know who it is, I can't tell who they are yet.

This has presented some problems because people are calling me now and saying "Hi Arlene. It's me!" which isn't a very helpful introduction. I think people assume that I will recognize their voices on the phone, but all voices tend to sound the same and I can't really distinguish between them. Another problem is that I haven't heard what people's voices sound like, even in person, for quite some time, many years in fact. So even if I heard them accurately, I still wouldn't know who they are. I have CallerID on my phone line, and even though so many calls come up as "unavailable" or "anonymous" on this box, at least it helps me figure out who some of those "Hi, it's me" people are.

I had to call for some airline flight arrival information and also to stop my newspaper delivery. Both these calls were handled by voice mail menus. I still get a kick out of the idea that voice mail menus are not hard for me, even though this often requires getting all the menu categories the first time, no second chances. I used to struggle with them, dialing into the recorded message again and again, but understanding them was virtually hopeless. I don't know how I am understanding these things now, but I can — I really can. I'm also finding that the phone numbers with recorded messages are fun to experiment with since they don't involve live people with limited patience. That's another thing I like about them. It's just me, my electronics and their electronics — no other human element, no commentary on how I am doing. If I need a repeat, I can always "press one" again.

These phone menus are part of our culture, something everyone knows about. But for me they are new. So again, I feel a bit like an alien landing on this planet — and also like a child, playing with my new toy.

DAY 64
FEBRUARY 2

I still find myself happily surprised when I hear things that I don't expect. The little pleasantries of life are just that — pleasant. The postal clerk who took my "hold mail" form said, "Terrific. Enjoy!" The toll collector said to have a nice day. The salesperson at an art gallery asked me if I had any questions. The cashier at the parking garage commented about the weather.

In each of these circumstances, without my CI, not only would I have missed out on those little words of sunshine, I would have been at a total loss, wondering if I was missing out on essential information. The postal clerk could have been asking me for additional information. The salesperson might have been telling me about new merchandise coming in. The parking garage cashier could have been asking me if I wanted a receipt. The toll collector might have been telling me something was wrong with my car. I wouldn't have known and I would have had to determine if it was worth the effort to try and find out what they were saying. Most of the time, I would have just put on my "all purpose" smile and hoped for the best. But that smile was always a joyless smile, a nervous reaction to not knowing what was going on around me.

This must sound trivial to people who have been told to "have a nice day" ad nauseam. But it is still new and fresh for me. Considering where I have come from, I don't think I am going to get tired of this any time soon.

I'm also getting the hang of the cosmetics of my speech processor. In the cold weather of the north, sweaters, jackets and vests easily conceal the unit. It's as if I don't have a choice in the matter — the realities of winter dressing make decision-making about concealing moot. In warmer climates or seasons, where there is less clothing, and some of that normally gets tucked in, there is a decision to be made — to conceal or not.

I had thought that I would want to conceal the speech processor, for two reasons — not to look too bulky and not to invite questions. At first, this was what I did, but it turned out to be impractical. So I tucked my tops in, and clipped the speech processor in its protective case to my belt. I thought I would feel kind of conspicuous about this arrangement, toting along excess baggage that other people don't need.

To my surprise and delight, that is not what happened at all! As I survey the crowds wherever I go, *everyone* has things clipped to their belts! Most of them are beepers, which are smaller than my speech processor. But some are cellular phones, which are usually at least as big and sometimes even larger. So instead of feeling self-conscious, as I expected to, I sort of swagger importantly now with a "can't leave home without my essential electronics" air.

DAY 70
FEBRUARY 8

I went to another captioned Broadway show yesterday, *Bring In Da Noise, Bring In Da Funk* and had a great time, once again. I had expected to check out how I was doing with the infrared system, curious if I would be able to understand the dialogue this time. It turns out this was the wrong show to judge that for. It was almost entirely tap dancing, with scat singing, rap and Black dialect for dialogue. I think everyone, hearing or not, appreciated the captioning for this show. I'm not disappointed about this because I had a wonderful experience that I didn't expect: I heard the marvelous sound of tap dancing, the intricate rhythms and beats that characterize this unique dance form.

The infrared system brought the singers' voices right into my "ears." I could also hear the crisp and distinct clicking of the dancers' feet. My mind wandered, thinking why I was enjoying this particular sound so much. Your senses have associations with the past, and this tapping sound brought me back to my own dancing school days at the Third Street Music School Settlement House. The settlement houses in lower Manhattan in the 1950's fielded some exceptionally talented faculty and my class was taught by José Limón, the founder of the José Limón Dance Company, a well-known dance troupe. We were taught modern dance, learning to leap and sway gracefully to music. I guess I should have felt privileged to have had this experience, but I was always a bit envious of the ballet classes on pointe, with ballet shoes, that my friends had. I was even more intrigued with tap dancing — and tap shoes. Modern dance required no shoes at all since we always danced barefoot — not very glamorous, especially to an eight-year-old.

I guess this latent desire stayed with me because about ten years ago, when I saw that the local Community School was offering Beginning Tap Dancing, I literally jumped at the chance. I took the first session, finally owning a pair of shiny black tap shoes. I loved the classes, and decided to sign up for the next session. But I was having a hard time hearing the beat of the music, so that is where my tap dancing career ended. I could "Shuffle Off To Buffalo," but I guess I wasn't destined to go any further.

About two years ago, I noticed that my regular shoes no longer made any noise when I walked on the kitchen floor. I tried a few "shuffle" tap steps, but heard nothing. In exactly the same location in the kitchen where my keys had stopped jingling years before, my feet stopped tapping. I think I should put a plaque up there.

The silence of my feet was disturbing enough, but I could no longer hear Shirley Temple tapping with Buddy Ebsen and Bo Jangles in the old movie reruns either. Ironically, many of those old movies were finally captioned, so I was able to understand them. Watching tap dancing in silence, though, leaves something to be desired, and that something is the click-click-click of those tap shoes. I had to cross yet another little pleasure off the list of things I enjoyed, another casualty of my hearing loss.

Can you imagine my delight at hearing all that tapping yesterday with my CI? Such an insignificant part of the universe, tap dancing — and yet, I loved it, I've always loved it, and I never get tired of watching it or listening to it. Yesterday's tapping was quintessential tap dancing — complicated rhythms spelled out by talented feet. Almost two hours of it, and I relished every minute.

DAY 73
FEBRUARY 11

I had another mapping session, nine weeks since getting my speech processor and only two weeks since my last one. My last appointment had been impromptu since I felt that I wasn't doing well with the programs I had. I thought I might cancel this appointment since it was so close to the last one, but my current programs weren't working that well for me, so I thought I would try for something better. It turns out I was right; my "numbers" had shifted again. My audiologist always tests for the threshold and comfort levels, and that's where we started this mapping session once again. My threshold levels have stayed pretty much the same, but my comfort levels had increased, and that is probably why I sensed that I needed a change. Everything had also started to take on a hazy quality and I wanted to try to get rid of that as well.

With the new threshold and comfort levels, we tried some new programs. I ended up getting one with noise suppression, one that had nothing cut out of it, and another that we had fine-tuned to sound the most natural. Sometimes the most natural-sounding isn't the best one for understanding speech, but it's worth giving it a try. We checked if I could still understand sentences without looking, which I could. I then had to decide whether to keep any of the old programs, so we compared the old program I had liked best with the new programs. The old one sounded tinny and thin in comparison, so again, throwing caution to the winds, I walked out with three new programs.

Back outside with the traffic noise of Manhattan, I flipped to the noise suppression program and that was fine. My next stop was the League for the Hard of Hearing, for an evaluation to see if I needed any aural rehabilitation with my CI. This had been suggested by my audiologist, and waiting until I had reached the two-month mark gave me sufficient time to get used to the speech processor.

I should mention that my adjustment to the sound provided by my CI has been very rapid. Not everyone's progress is this fast. People who are either prelingually deafened, have been deaf for a long time, or have always had a hearing loss would not expect the same rapid adaptation as someone who has lost her hearing later in life. Rehabilitation is suggested for all CI users, no matter how they are doing, so that the person can make optimal use of the sounds being transmitted by the speech processor. The appropriate type of rehabilitation is determined by assessing how well speech can be understood.

At my evaluation, Pat Rothschild, Director of the Communication Department, conversed with me first. "Conversed" is an understatement here. Pat was my first speechreading teacher at the League for the Hard of Hearing, so we go "way back." ("Speechreading" refers to using all visual cues, not just the lips, to discern speech. I use the term interchangeably with "lipreading.") This evaluation gave us a grand opportunity to catch up on old times, but with an ironic twist. During our classes together, I had been trained to concentrate on her face and lip movements as she "spoke" with no voice. At this evaluation, I had to listen to her voice, with her face totally blocked by a cloth screen. My brain started talking to me again. "Can't you make up your mind what you want me to do? First you train me to watch her mouth closely, and now you're telling me to forget all that?!" Yes, brain, you've got it right. Just listen.

I had to repeat one-syllable words, both face-to-face and on the phone. The words all started and ended with a consonant. By analyzing my responses, we could tell if I was having any trouble with particular speech sounds. I got most of the sounds, but we found that I was confusing the "k" sound and the "p" sound, saying "patch" for "catch" and vice versa. I was also mixing up the "s" and "f" sound over the phone. This error didn't surprise me at all. Invariably, when my name and address are given over the phone,

I receive mail addressed to "Arlene Romoss." So mixing up these two sounds over the phone seems to be "normal." I then had to repeat sentences back from a story as they were read to me (without looking, of course). I was able to do this with only a few minor errors. This was all very good news. The only bad news was that I couldn't hear the phone ring. I guess my "noise suppression" got carried away.

From this evaluation, we decided that there wasn't anything in particular that I needed to work on. I could bear in mind which sounds I might confuse, but in context I probably wouldn't have a problem with them. Pat suggested I listen to books on tape, which I knew to be standard advice to anyone with a CI. The idea of listening to books that I had always wanted to read, but had never gotten around to, sounded very appealing. My brain still goes into a panic when it is forced to listen to speech without visual cues ("The mouth! The mouth! Where's the mouth?"), strongly conditioned over the years. So this listening plan should help calm things up there as well.

I've been using the new programs for two days now, and they are really better than the old ones. This is the first time that a new mapping has made a noticeable difference. I usually listen to some audio speech on my computer where the dialogue has always been difficult to understand. Sometimes I could only pick up words here and there, missing most of it. With the new programs, I can get more of the words, not clearly, but with concentration, they are coming in better. I also noticed that I was doing better understanding television dialogue, even on the large-screen tv, which I have to view at a distance. I still use the captions, though, switching back and forth between following along with the words and listening only. I'm also hearing greater nuances in the sounds around me, which is encouraging. My next appointment is in a month, my three-month evaluation, so I have some time to "fiddle" and "grow" with these programs. They look promising so far.

DAY 85
FEBRUARY 23

It's been exactly 12 weeks since I began using my speech processor. My last mapping was two weeks ago, and my initial impressions about it were correct. I am doing better with it than with previous mappings. I have changed over the last two weeks, just as I had changed after previous mappings. I started out preferring the program that had noise control on it, finding the programs with no noise control uncomfortable except in the quietest of surroundings. That has changed, and now the program that has no noise control is my favorite. The program that was supposed to make voices sound most natural doesn't. The one that doesn't "shape" the sound at all does. Go figure!

I am getting better at this. My confidence in my hearing is building gradually and I sense that this hearing is starting to belong to me. Before getting my CI, I could always count on losing hearing, sometimes noticeably so, in a span of three months. So it is unusual to experience an improvement in hearing in that amount of time.

Everyone told me that things would continue to get "better," but nobody ever really said "how." There is so much involved in hearing. I do get the feeling now that everything is getting "better" — phone use, understanding without looking, music, hearing in noise. As I've said before, I've been turning back the clock. There's nothing I am more familiar with than every little step of the way from normal hearing to profound deafness. It took me almost 30 years to do that (talk about learning the hard way!), so I have a very good perspective on what I might expect going the other way, getting my hearing back. After all, 30 years is a long time to study any subject, especially if you are the guinea pig.

So what does it mean to say I'm doing "better?" Some concrete criteria come to mind. To begin with, visualize the ability to hear as three categories — Level 1, 2, and 3, or, in Olympics terms, Gold, Silver and Bronze. At the Gold level, you are able to comprehend speech without looking and you are able to understand it instantly without thinking about it. Hear — understand. That is the best hearing.

At the Silver level, you comprehend speech, but have to concentrate to understand the words. Since you have to use the initial mental process just to comprehend the words, it requires another process to interpret what those words mean. An example of this is when you hear on the phone, but have to concentrate on what people are saying, figure out what they mean, and then respond. At this level of hearing, because you first have to field the words, it is harder to "think on your feet." The listening process has been slowed down. Hear — process — understand.

This level is also the first inkling that something is wrong when you start to lose your hearing. People may accuse you of not paying attention or not listening. You start to feel that maybe it is your fault that you can't catch everything, that if only you tried a little harder, you would be able to hear better. This is probably the root of "bluffing," pretending to hear even if you don't. On the way down, Silver hearing is baffling, to have to think to hear. On the way back, Silver hearing is terrific. "Wow — imagine being able to hear without looking! So what if I have to concentrate!" It's all a matter of perspective, I guess.

At the Bronze level, you can hear the words, but you can't understand what they are. Hear — process — process — process — process — nada. But there is more to comprehending speech than by hearing alone. If you add visual cues, by lipreading and body language, then comprehension can be greatly improved. Adding visual cues at the Silver level, for example, often fools the brain into thinking that it is really hearing at the Gold level. There is no need to process the sound because the visuals make up for the lack of clarity. At the Bronze level, visual cues are extremely important because there would be no speech comprehension without them.

Let's say that you are hearing almost everything — 90% hearing and 10% visual cues. Lipreading at this level would be very easy to do. You would get total speech comprehension, and you probably wouldn't have to process that sound. Your brain would get the content instantly, like the Gold level. Hear/see — understand. What happens with less and less sound is that you have to lipread more and more. The more lipreading you need to do, the more the brain has to process that information. The better the lipreader, the less dependent on the amount of sound. Without any sound, only about 30% of speech movements are visible, which makes comprehension extremely difficult even for the best lipreaders. Everyone is different, but in my case, I would say that if I am lipreading up to about 50%, I can do it fluently: hear/see — understand. At 60% lipreading, I'm still okay, although I would probably have to process at that level: hear/see — process — understand, and I would only be able to function one-on-one like that. At over 70% lipreading, things start to slow down. Not only would I have to speak to one person at a time, I would also have to be told the topic and which person is talking. Right before I got my CI, I was hearing less than 10% and lipreading over 90%. I was not functioning well at that level, I was under constant stress, and it was making me miserable.

At this Bronze level, where visual cues are still necessary, the CI helps a *lot*, bringing in consonant sounds to make lipreading so much easier. That is what is so important about the CI — even if I can't always understand without looking, I am able to function much more effectively with visual cues. There's also a greater likelihood that I wouldn't be restricted to one-on-one conversations, and that I could get enough sound so I wouldn't have to "process" the words. My brain would understand without that extra step.

Now that you have an idea of how even *some* extra sound can help, there are actually four situations I find myself in that contribute to how well I'm doing with my CI: quiet/close-up, noise/close-up, quiet/far and noise/far.

	/ noise	/ quiet
close	x	x
far	x	x

There! I always wanted to do that! It's a graphic illustration of the ways in which I can do "better." When I first got my CI, I did incredibly well, being able to repeat sentences up close and in quiet, without looking. I was either lucky, or whatever combination of hearing history, equipment and luck contributed to that success. But even though I could repeat the sentences without looking, it was Silver hearing, not Gold. I was really working at it, the way you would squint your eyes to see things better in focus. That first day with my CI, when I was listening to Ira talk to me in the car, without looking — it was Silver hearing. I could do it, but I was concentrating hard. Similarly, with the phone, although I could use it after a week with my CI, it was Silver hearing.

Now, I can hear Ira, up close and in quiet, without having to think. (I also can tell you what he is going to say before he says it, but that has more to do with our being married almost 28 years, than my CI.) The phone is becoming easier, and last week, I was even able to complete a phone call that required me to "think on my feet." I felt for the first time that I wasn't using all my thought processes to hear the words. I still had some energy left to formulate a response.

I'm able to hear better in noise up close. A good illustration is a noisy restaurant with some background music. We were in that situation last week and I was able to flip to my "noise suppression" program and also to set the sensitivity down to block out a lot of the background noise. I think I have also started to block out some background noise on my own. I was able to continue having a conversation at least one-on-one in this environment. I was fielding enough sound in this "Bronze" situation to be able to lipread without much difficulty. What is interesting is that in this environment, sometimes *hearing* people can't function. There is too much noise for them to utilize their normal Gold or even Silver hearing, so they are thrust into the Bronze area, yet they have few lipreading skills to function there. Some hearing people are really annoyed by this — that supposedly "hearing impaired" people can function in an environment where hearing people can't. There is something to be said for bionics and 30 years spent perfecting lipreading skills!

Hearing from a distance, like loudspeaker announcements, also seems to be improving. I heard raffle numbers being called over a public address system this past weekend. That surprised me! Hearing the television from across the room is still eluding me, though. Some television programs come in better than others, but I'm able to follow along with the captions easily.

There's one other category that can get "better" and that is music. With this last mapping, my piano is sounding a little bit more like a piano although still somewhat electronic. I'm finding that for listening to the piano, radio or recorded speech, turning the sensitivity setting all the way down makes things sound more natural. I'm still dabbling with this, knowing full well that my own perception of these sounds is still changing.

So there, in a very large nutshell, is what it means to hear "better." Everyone's experience with a CI is unique, but no matter how one does at the beginning, we all experience doing "better" over time.

DAY 86
FEBRUARY 24

I was thinking about what I wrote yesterday, explaining how I'm hearing with this CI and how I'm improving. Sometimes writing about my experiences reveals thoughts I didn't know I had. I wrote that now I am getting the feeling that I own this hearing, something I hadn't felt before. It has all been so new — I had been concentrating on what was different, what had changed in my life. But as time goes on, this is my life; this hearing is now my hearing. It is now almost three months old and as it becomes my hearing, I am using it as if I've always had it. Maybe I'm becoming convinced that this isn't a temporary gift.

I once had a temporary gift of hearing 24 years ago. I was pregnant with my first child, and somewhere around the middle of my sixth month, my hearing suddenly returned. At that time, I had a moderate hearing loss and, with this unexpected boost, I found that I was hearing better without my hearing aid! A quick hearing test confirmed this assessment. That utopian existence lasted two weeks, and as quickly as it came, it departed. Nothing as dramatic ever happened again, not even during my next pregnancy. You can understand that I am a little hesitant to embrace my new hearing unconditionally just yet. But with each passing day, then week, then month, I am starting to be convinced that this is now "my hearing" and the past is just that — history.

Today was a case in point. I had a doctor's appointment and errands to run — nothing exciting, but as I moved through the day, it was exciting. I found myself doing ordinary things with a fresh vigor — with no fear, with no deaf ball and chain to drag me down.

The doctor's visit was my first, for myself, since getting my speech processor. I had taken my mother to the doctor last week and the experience there was exactly the same as today's visit. I didn't have to worry about hearing the doctor. I could concentrate on health issues, not hearing. This was the first time in an age that I had been able to do that. From hearing the nurse telling me what to do, to consulting with the doctor in his office, we were not talking about hearing, about facing me when you speak, about positioning microphones, about hearing hearing hearing. Aside from the medical aspects of my implant, hearing had nothing to do with our discussions. It was just the way it should be — at last. Normal.

I had a prescription to fill and even that was a refreshing activity. The pharmacist was asking me questions from his balcony perch; you know the way pharmacies are laid out. I couldn't understand him at that distance without looking so I asked him to please repeat. Once I was looking at him, I could understand him fine. When he came down to the front counter, I had no trouble hearing him, and I'm not even sure if I was looking at him or not. It didn't seem to matter at close range. He was telling me that one prescription would be ready later, and he would call me. I didn't have to explain about Relay or how to use it. I didn't have to worry about getting a phone call, wondering whether it was going to be Relay or not. (Even recalling this process is making me nervous!) I just gave him my phone number and said, "Call me." No explanations, no problems — no sweat! Normal.

I was starting to feel very happy. Two tasks down so far and I was flying! Free to be me, no "hearing" baggage to tote around. Next stop was the shopping mall to pick up some sundries. I completed that mission and was heading for the exit when I passed a Bell Atlantic Mobile cellular phone display in the middle of the mall. I had always looked at those booths, sadly acknowledging that they were not for me. It had become such a habit, I almost passed it again. But wait! I can hear on a regular phone now. I can hear sales people now. So I went up to the booth, wanting to know what they had to offer. I told the salesman I needed a hearing aid-compatible phone (because when I mentioned cochlear implant, he had no idea what I was talking about.) He hadn't a clue about hearing aid-compatible phones either. So I told him I needed a phone that didn't cause interference when I held it up to my device. He suggested one model and I tried it — and I heard with it. It wasn't great because I didn't want to reset my speech processor, otherwise I wouldn't have heard the salesman optimally. I was just happy to be trying these phones out. I tried another one, but it stuck to the magnet of my headpiece, pulling it off my head. Nope, that wasn't going to be "the one." I tried another, and I heard on that. I must have looked like a real novice, trying to dial those little phones with the teensy pushbuttons. I was also having a hard time seeing the numbers without my reading glasses. Great — now that I can hear, I can't see! I thanked the salesman for his time, and told him I would have to think about my needs. Yes! I was just like the people I had watched for years and years, trying out those phones in the mall. Normal.

That episode made me even happier, so I decided to treat myself. I stopped at the Gap, daring to shop solo with no daughter to guide me. The music was bopping from above. Most of the stores have music and I've come to expect it. The rhythm and basic beat came through fine even though I couldn't hear much else. In this great mood, I was practically dancing around the store, picking out shirts and skirts to try on. This time I could understand the marketing strategy, and the marketing experts would have been proud. I was having the enjoyable shopping experience they were counting on. As I danced my purchases to the cashier, I happily acknowledged the clerk's "nice day" wishes, and headed out the door. Normal.

With the hearing that I can now claim as mine, I'm able to do so many things that hearing people can. It's still going to take me a little more time to get used to this, but I don't feel like an outsider anymore. I'm starting to feel normal.

DAY 87
FEBRUARY 25

A funny thing happened to me today. I met an acquaintance I hadn't seen in a year. She was a little perplexed because she thought she knew who I was, but the person she was thinking of had always struggled to understand her. The person in front of her was calm, conversing easily, and having no trouble understanding. Was I that same person?

What could I say? Yes, I'm the person she thought I was; that much I could tell her. But am I the same person — the one who had to struggle to hear, the one who could neither hold a casual conversation with an acquaintance, nor wanted to? No, she really hadn't met me before. She had met a person trapped in a prison of silence, unable to "be herself." The smiling person having the free-flowing conversation was me and if you've never had that sort of conversation with me, then I guess you've never really met "me."

We're still trying to see a movie that I can hear and enjoy. It's been so frustrating, bringing along my infrared equipment, and not having the systems work right. We tried again this past weekend to see As Good As It Gets. Our strategy this time was for Ira to get a headset and test it out, figuring that if it worked for him, my receiver should work for me. We got a big bag of popcorn and a soda, and we settled into seats towards the front, closest to a speaker in the ceiling. We figured that if the infrared didn't work, at least I would be closer to the sound source. (And if I couldn't hear, at least I could eat!) The infrared didn't work, at least not very well. Ira said it had a f-f-f-f-f sound to it, not a strong signal. I tried mine anyway, but couldn't pick up any signal either. It was on, but not transmitting any sound. Sigh.

I watched the movie as best I could and after about a half hour, the battery on my speech processor died. (Popcorn must drain those batteries!) I quickly replaced it and realized that I was hearing a little better with the new battery — about half the dialogue. I guess the battery must lose a slight amount of power right before it dies, but I never noticed it before. This hearing situation was marginal, though. I was at a distance from the speaker, which is more difficult for me, and I couldn't lipread all the actors because they weren't always facing front.

As Good As It Gets never got very good although other people had thought so, including the critics. Maybe the fewer movies you've seen in your life, the more picky you become. As the credits were scrolling and we walked up the aisle to exit the theater, Ira thought he'd try the headset one more time from the back. He put it on — and, lo and behold, the signal was strong! He told me, "Quick, plug your receiver in!" I plugged in right away, but still nothing. Then we realized that the receiver he had was a regular headphone shape, with the receiver button on top, and since the signal was strong in the rear of the theater, that was probably where the infrared signal was coming from. A lightbulb went on in my head, "Turn your receiver around, dummy. Face it to the back of the theater!" I did that — and — SOUND! I caught the very last chords of the credit-scrolling music.

Now it all made sense. This was the same system that I had tried without success in the movie theater in Florida, where they gave out the same Martian-looking headphones. I'll bet they were beaming it from the rear there also. People who take these headphones should be aware of that. And people who bring their own receivers to plug into their CI speech processors or hearing aids should be aware that they may have to point the receiver backwards, something that defies common sense. Who in their right mind would put on a receiver and then point it backwards?! From now on, in movie theaters that give out Martian headphones — ME!

DAY 90
FEBRUARY 28

Yesterday, I attended my synagogue for the first time since getting my CI. The sanctuary is equipped with an infrared listening system and I feel largely responsible for its being there. When we moved to the area 14 years ago and joined the temple, it became apparent that I couldn't hear in that large sanctuary with its high, vaulted ceilings, even with my hearing aid. I spoke to the Rabbi about installing an assistive listening system. He said that the temple was already considering it, but had never acted on it. I remember his words exactly, though. He said, "If one person in this congregation needs it, then we should have it." That was pre-ADA, and religious institutions are not bound by the ADA anyway, but they do answer to a higher authority.

The infrared system was put in and I remember distinctly the very first day I used it there. I could hear the Rabbi perfectly — 100% without looking, better than with my hearing aid. I heard the tinkle of the tiny silver bells on the Torah decorations as they were taken out of the Ark. It was a miracle — a true miracle — as I explained to everyone how somehow the sound was picked up by the microphones, turned into invisible infrared light, beamed out to the congregation, picked up by the individual receivers, and then somehow turned back into sound.

It was a miracle that first year, and even the second and third. But as my hearing continued to decline, I could no longer hear 100% with it, so it became a lipreading aid. Little by little, I heard less and less, and lipread more and more. By the High Holy Days last fall, it was pointless to listen with the system at all because it gave me no usable sound. The system still worked, but not for me any longer.

I attended the Yizkor memorial service at that time. Aside from saying Kaddish for my father, who had passed away in March, I also wanted to hear the Rabbi recite the names of those who had died in the past year. I knew I wouldn't be able to hear my father's name being called, but a memorial booklet listed the names in order, and Ira pointed out each one as the Rabbi recited them. When he came to my father's name, I looked up so I could at least lipread the Rabbi as he said it. Emanuel M. Klinger. I saw it being mouthed. I worked so hard just to see that name spoken.

Yesterday, I attended the Friday night service because it was my father's Yahrzeit, the anniversary of his death one year ago. I came to say Kaddish for him and again to hear the Rabbi read his name aloud, along with the names of others who had passed away at this time in years past.

I used the infrared system and I was all set with the proper cord and receiver, positioned (not backwards) to get an optimal signal. As the Rabbi spoke and the Cantor sang, I adjusted the volume and sensitivity settings — and I was back! It was almost like connecting the first time, 14 years before! Not quite. The music was not as good, but the speech was crisp and clear. I didn't test myself to see if I could understand without looking. I was content to follow along in the prayer book and to watch the Rabbi as he addressed the congregation.

At the Kaddish portion of the service, I waited for the Rabbi to announce my father's name. This time, there was no printed list. I would have to follow on my own. I heard each name, in alphabetical order. And then I heard the name I had been waiting for — Emanuel M. Klinger. I heard it.

A theological question was discussed: if you know the scientific reasoning behind a "miracle," is it still a miracle? We were, of course, referring to my miracle, enabling the deaf to hear. I described the process which allowed me to hear the Rabbi. His voice was picked up by the microphone, which fed it to the sound system, which was attached to the infrared transmitter, which converted it to light, which the infrared receiver converted back into sound, which was then fed into my speech processor, which processed the sound, sending the signal to the computer chip under my scalp, which fired the electrodes thousands of times per second in my cochlea, which stimulated my auditory nerve, which let my brain hear the Rabbi's words. All of this occurred so quickly that the lip movements I saw were perfectly synchronized with what I heard.

You could say that it is a miracle that scientists could perfect such technology. That may be true, but why should this be possible at all? And if this is not a miracle, what is?

DAY 96
MARCH 6

I was going to say the honeymoon is over, now that I've had my CI for three months, but, really, it's the trial period that's over. I'm not giving it back — no way, no how! This hearing is now becoming mine and I'm using it as if it is mine, not testing it out so much. I'm starting to move about differently, with more confidence. I answer the phone anywhere in the house without running to the kitchen line to check the Caller ID. Anyway, most of the time, the Caller ID box says "anonymous," "no data sent," or "unavailable." They have so many ways to tell you this little box is useless! I finally took the hint and was courageous enough to pick up any phone and say "hello." Understanding the names on the other end takes some concentration, but I've been able to manage. The repeat callers are getting better about identifying themselves, as I've had to ask even close friends and relatives, "Who am I speaking with?"

Of course, I've been introduced to the world of telemarketers. I had always answered the phone, even when I barely had any hearing left. I would try to tell if a Relay call was coming in by straining to hear the words "TTY user." Relay operators always announced that they had "a Relay call for a TTY user." I had to figure out if the call was a telemarketer, and it always seemed a shame to put so much stress, struggle and energy into a computer-generated or rote call, but that comes with the territory of not hearing. The worst calls were the telemarketers who pretended they knew you, or were your friend. "How are you today?" they'd ask. They were making chitchat while I had no idea what they were saying, all the time straining to hear the words "TTY user." I would automatically tell whoever was on the line to call me back by Relay if I didn't hear those golden words, "TTY user." Occasionally, I even told Relay operators to call me back by Relay. . . .

Mercifully, telemarketers wouldn't usually call back by Relay. In the seven years that I used Relay, it only happened twice. They must have been very desperate (or nice — I don't know which). I felt obligated at least to chat with them and thank them for calling me back, but I was never grateful enough to actually *buy* something from them.

This struggle is now over. What's new to me is that I'm discovering what kinds of businesses have been calling me all these years. In the span of a week, I have been approached by phone solicitors for *Golf for Women* magazine, roofing and siding, the Salvation Army, equity loans, refinancing my home, carpet and upholstery cleaning, AT&T Visa card, a New York City survey, and an alarm system. Regular voice phone users probably see this as no big deal, a typical nuisance. But for years, these telemarketing calls had been a *special* nuisance for me because I couldn't tell them from regular calls or if they were something truly important. I did develop a nonchalant attitude eventually, thinking that if they didn't call back by Relay, it couldn't have been important. But I always wondered. Now, I know.

As they say, don't get mad, get even, so now I use these callers for telephone practice. Stress-free practice. I've detected a rhythm to their spiels, too. There are slight pauses where they almost expect you to tell them, "No," or even to hang up. I can tell you that by staying on the line, you encourage them. I listened to an entire sales promotion for an alarm system, and when I finally told them I wasn't interested, they wouldn't believe me. They assumed they were practically at my house, in my door. "Sorry," I thought, with a smug little smile. "You didn't call me back by Relay all those years. I'm making up for some lost time."

DAY 98
MARCH 8

I've been having doubts whether I could last until my next mapping since sounds seemed to be changing almost daily. A hoarse quality was coming in. I thought it was going to get worse, but it hasn't. It's either better or I've gotten used to it, probably a combination. I will do some adjusting in my mapping tomorrow, but it's not making me crazy.

This is the first time I've felt that I really want to save a program, rather than chuck them all and explore uncharted territory. Of the three programs, I'm only using the flat one, the one with nothing done to it, no shaping of sound or noise suppression. I either outgrew the other programs or they are just wrong for me now. The noise suppression program is suppressing too much and even in noisy situations, it's not better than my flat program. The third program, the one which was supposed to make things sound more natural, lost this race at the starting line. Out in the real world, it didn't sound any better than the flat program, and sometimes worse. I kept checking to see if it would come around, but it is really useless. So that leaves the flat program, which I am doing nicely with. I've had it about four weeks. It was good in the beginning, and it's even better now.

I finally took out audio tapes from the library. I've been sort of slow in that department. My local library had a nice selection, but nothing I was looking for. I thought I'd take out some classics that I had never read, but they had mostly best sellers and non-fiction self-improvement tapes, with only a few titles I would consider "classic." And almost all the tapes available were abridged versions. The conventional wisdom is to take out the tape and follow along with the book. You can't do that with an abridged version. Oh well, I thought, switch to Plan B. We'll give them a try anyway, even if there is no book to follow along with.

I also meant to buy a Walkman tape player, but since I haven't done that yet, I figured I'd try a cassette in my car's tape player. I've been listening to the news and weather without too much difficulty, so I didn't think I was setting myself up for disaster. I plunked it in, and — fine! As a matter of fact, it was so fine that I didn't want to get out of my car. Fortunately, the ride to visit my mother is almost two hours each way, so that gave me plenty of time. Listening is supposed to get you used to hearing spoken language, so I was getting a mighty big dose of it traveling to my mother.

I found I could understand the self-help tapes in the car although at high speeds, the road noise made it more difficult. These were narrated with a consistent voice level, but the fiction was dramatized. When the volume of the voices varies a lot, it's too hard for me to understand in the car, especially with the road noise. I got an instant education in how to work my car's sound system, though. My cars had always had cassette and CD players, but I never used them. I had never even played with the buttons before, so it was a feat just getting to the beginning of the tapes. I could have read the manual, of course, but that would have been too easy.

I figured out how to fast forward, rewind, play, reverse, eject — all while driving the car! I got pretty good at rewinding and replaying what I couldn't understand. The controls on my car stereo are easy to use and I'm fortunate that this system is top quality. It's like being in my own sound cubicle, where I can adjust the volume to my own needs, and it works very well for me. So now I'm all "self-helped," having listened to over six hours of this stuff. I've learned how to negotiate anything, and I'm on my way to honing the proper habits of a highly effective person. The thing I could really use is a tape to teach me how to remember all this!

Listening to fiction in the car was proving to be too difficult. The road noise was drowning out the *sotto voces*, so that made me decide to get my act together and buy myself a Walkman tape player. I bought a Sony Walkman with digital tuning and when I got it home, I dropped in the tape of *The Secret Garden*. I already had the patch cord, which I had been using to connect my speech processor to my infrared receiver, and it worked for the Walkman too. By plugging the Walkman straight into my speech processor, there was no background noise, so the sound came in much clearer than listening to it in the car. It was narrated by a woman with a British accent who was not easy to understand, but I made my way through it, rewinding and replaying when necessary.

This was the first time I had ever listened to fiction on tape. Now that I think about it, I must have always had some sort of speech discrimination problem, long before I noticed it. I remember in my high school sophomore English class having a difficult time following a recording of Dickens. I recall being able to hear it, but having to concentrate very hard on the words. Remember my "Silver" hearing definition, having to concentrate to understand? That was probably the beginning of my hearing decline. So for me to be able to listen to spoken English, and understand it — this was really a first for me. I never did it before nor wanted to. Now I do.

All three tapes went back to the library and I was eager to get more. I think I'm getting hooked on this. Now that I knew I really could hear them, I scoured the selections more carefully. I took out Alan Dershowitz's *Chutzpah* and Russell Baker's memoirs. On the trip back from the library, in went the Dershowitz tape. I didn't really know what to expect. Now I know. *Chutzpah* is his perspective on Jews and anti-Semitism, and it is narrated by Dershowitz himself. I listened to it, rapt, fascinated not only by the text, but also with the idea of hearing the author's own voice. Like listening to a composer play his own concerto, it was a powerful way to "read" a book, far more interesting than scanning pages of written text visually.

These thoughts brought back memories of a "performance" I had heard many many years ago. Ira and I had attended an antique show in an armory and there was a dealer selling Steinway grand pianos with a built-in player piano mechanism. The music made by this machine sounded so magnificent, it was hard to believe that all that shading and emotion could be produced from air blowing though holes in a paper roll. What was I listening to that could possibly have been so memorable? George Gershwin was playing a piano arrangement of *Rhapsody in Blue*, reproduced on this six-foot Steinway grand piano and filling the armory with an

explosion of sound. Gershwin himself had originally played it on a recording piano to produce the paper roll. Like the "Phantom of the Armory," the
keys bounced up and down, as if he was actually striking them. This was not
a recording. It was Gershwin playing Gershwin on a Steinway grand. And
now I was listening to Dershowitz reading Dershowitz. Maybe not as exciting as the Gershwin experience, but powerful all the same.

Again, I didn't want to get out of the car. I had intended to leave
one tape in the car and listen to the harder ones on the Walkman at
home. So much for plans. I couldn't wait. I took the tape out of the car and
brought it into the house to listen on my Walkman.

Now I'm hooked. I was anxious to start listening to the Russell
Baker tape, and put that in my car stereo on my next round of errands.
Again, I couldn't bring myself to turn the thing off. So I ejected it from my
car stereo and plunked it into my Walkman at home. This "audio therapy"
turned out to be a lot more interesting than I had anticipated. Once
inside, I started playing the Baker tape, but I looked at the time and
wondered when I would fit in the exercise walk I had planned. Sitting there
listening to tapes was therapeutic for my ears, but the rest of me needed
some help too! Then another lightbulb went off in my head, "This is a
Walkman, dummy, not a Sitman!"

I had never walked outside with a Walkman on although everyone
in the neighborhood does. "Now I can do that too," I thought. I wasn't quite
sure where to clip everything, but out I went with the Walkman plugged into
my speech processor, the speech processor clipped to my belt and the
Walkman in my hand. I thought that would make it easiest to rewind the
tape in case I missed any of the dialogue.

As soon as I got outside, I immediately realized that I was different
from all the other Walkman users I had ever seen. I didn't have headphones.
Everyone always has headphones. They are no use to me because my ears
are just for show now, elaborately-designed earring holders. I wasn't sure if
I was comfortable with all this yet — looking like a Walkman user, but not
appearing to have any way to hear it. So I put my hood on. I'm sure no one
would have noticed anything strange or unusual, but I felt better that
way. I was ready for my debut into the power-walking world of Walkmen!

I was deaf to the world again, but with extenuating circumstances. The thrill of crunching on acorns had lost its appeal. How soon we are jaded about life's delights! There weren't many acorns left anyway, I rationalized. It was March, and the squirrels had eaten most of them. Walking with the sounds of Mother Nature is nice, but, well, you know, the novelty had worn off. Around the block I went, all the while following Russell Baker's trials and tribulations in the newspaper world. I started to get tired before the tape was over. It was unrealistic of me to expect to last the entire length of the tape, three hours. I did walk far longer than I would have without the tape.

During my next car ride, I finished the tape, happy to know that this is a new part of my life (and content to hear that Mr. Baker was safely ensconced at the *New York Times*). The implications of listening to books on tape are incredible; all this dead time can now be used to fill up my head with facts and fancy. I haven't forgotten about listening to music or the news, but to be able to listen to books? So many hours have been spent in boring isolation in the car and on walks. Lost time, wasted time. I have some catching up to do.

I also got a chance to try some new CD's I bought a few days ago, listening to them in my car's CD player. I know they would sound better if I played them in a CD-man or whatever it is they call Walkman's CD-playing cousin, but I don't own one yet. The Chopin piano music doesn't sound too bad. I heard it as piano music, but it sounded sort of flat. It had dynamic range and I could tell the lower registers from the upper, but it lacked absolute pitch. And the tonal quality — well, instead of conjuring up an image of Arthur Rubinstein, I kept picturing Schroeder playing his heart out. I hope this improves with practice.

Bach organ music lasted about a minute in the stereo player. It sounded so bad I didn't want to listen to it. It must have some harmonics or something that just cannot be processed by the speech processor (why do you think they call it a "speech" processor?), or by my brain, at this stage. Big band music didn't sound much better, so that, too, will have to wait. Music that involves just one instrument, or one instrument and simple accompaniment seems to sound better. It's hard to generalize, so I will continue to try it all.

One last item. I was out running errands when my CI battery died. I always carry a spare battery or two, but this time I had neglected to refill and replenish. I was deaf again. I also wasn't far from home, so rather than try to complete my little missions deaf, I went home to reload my equipment. It was a humbling reminder that this coach turns into a pumpkin if you don't play by the rules.

DAY 101
MARCH 11

My three-month evaluation was two days ago. I didn't need to be told how I was doing, and whatever numbers came up to quantify my CI progress would be approximations anyway. I knew I could hear in some situations without looking, but not all — not by a long shot. And I knew I was starting to do better in noise. Distance still mattered, sometimes frustratingly so, but they don't test for that.

I found that I had no emotional attachment to this evaluation. As I sat there listening to sentences and words, I didn't feel as though I, personally, was being tested — certainly not in the same way regular hearing tests had tracked my own hearing loss over the years. Those tests were on my own ears, my original equipment. My three-month CI evaluation was measuring how well some sophisticated computer gadget was allowing me to hear. It's a peculiar distinction, but one that I'd like to explain further.

Taking a hearing test had always been a depressing ritual. For 30 years, the news was always bad — less hearing, less hearing, less hearing, less, less, less. With each successive test, I struggled to cling to the hearing I had. The word lists were the most trying, as each time I was able to repeat fewer and fewer words until I could understand none by hearing alone. I always came prepared with tissues, and used them. No amount of trying (or crying) could help, yet it always seemed that if I just tried a little harder, I should be able to understand those words. But I was wrong. The scores kept dropping — 95%, 80%, 75% — and then I stopped going for tests for a few years, seeing no point to this torture. When I started again, it was 40%, 25% — and then none.

We are so conditioned to test scores that a 40% or 25% were dismal failures, and try as I might not to take it personally, I always did. If you get a 40% on a test, you've failed. Intellectually, I understood it wasn't for lack of trying but, to me, it was more than that. My body had failed. I was no longer "perfect." I had to confront the words "disability," "handicap" and "deaf." This does not come easily and those hearing tests confirmed the reality I knew without being told.

Ironically, the only hearing test I enjoyed was the one to determine if I was a CI candidate. In that *Through the Looking Glass* world, bad news was good. Not hearing meant that I could at last harbor the hope that a CI would bring some hearing back. With each word I couldn't understand, I was happy, knowing that I was one step closer to getting my CI.

So this three-month CI evaluation was for "them," for "them" to see how well "their" equipment was allowing me to hear. I had done my best to use this equipment as instructed. Whatever I heard was a measure of how the equipment was working for me. I did not feel emotionally involved with the process, as I had with my own ears.

I used my current favorite program for the tests. A pure-tone test was first, then sentences in quiet, then in noise, and then one-syllable words. The pure-tone test showed that with this program, at the settings I used to converse in a quiet room, I had the hearing of a person with a mild hearing loss. It really doesn't mean that I function outside in the real world as someone with a mild loss, but I guess they have to establish some benchmark of hearing.

I did very well with the sentence tests, even in noise. I had felt that my hearing in noise had improved, and my impressions had proven correct. I had to really concentrate in the noise, but yes, I could pull in that male voice on the tape recording. The single-syllable words were more difficult and I had a harder time with them, but still did quite well. I heard over 98% of the sentences in quiet, over 95% of the sentences in noise, and over 70% of the one-syllable words. My pre-CI results were 8% of the sentences in quiet and zero for everything else.

When we got to the single-syllable words, something funny happened. I realized that when I repeated them, they sounded the same as what I was hearing. This wasn't what I had become accustomed to. I must have adapted to my declining hearing because I used to guess at a word, but when I said it, it wouldn't sound like what I heard. I don't even know why I guessed at a particular word. All I can think of is that my brain had recalibrated what I heard, so if I heard "oh," it could recognize it as "boat" (or at least guess at it) even with a lot of the sounds missing. But when I said the word "boat," it didn't sound the same as the word I had heard. My brain had been trying to make the best of a bad situation, almost creating a new language based on what I could still hear. This may account for some of my initial success with the CI, being able to recognize words even from incomplete speech sounds.

Next was my mapping session. Some of my thresholds and comfort levels had shifted. I knew I wanted to keep one program, the one I had just been tested with, a flat program. We put that one in my speech processor, and another flat one too, that used the new, more powerful levels.

I had not been using my "noise" program at all, as I was quite successful in noise with my old flat program, so we felt that noisy situations were "covered." Then we dabbled, trying different things. We tried boosting trebles (too shrill), taking out middles (that had possibilities), but settled on something a little "quirkier," a program that doesn't fire the electrodes in ascending (or descending) order, but randomly. Why that should sound different is beyond me, but it did, and that too looked promising.

After using all three programs, sometimes I find that one is better than another. The sands are still shifting, so I'm still fiddling as I adapt to them. (It usually takes at least a week.) But the Chopin piano CD I listened to in my car definitely sounds better with the "scrambled" program — less electronic, more like a piano. It's still not great, but holds out possibilities. And that "scrambled" program also seems to pull in voices better in noise, but it is not always better — again, trial and error, error and trial. I won't go back for a remapping until June unless I'm having problems, and I won't have another evaluation until my one-year anniversary. So I continue to rejoice, hearing speech in quiet, but continuing to work on noise, distance and music.

DAY 104
MARCH 14

I've been dabbling with these new programs for a few days now and the jury is still out. I've been to meetings, used them with an infrared receiver at a show, with the phone, as well as in normal conversation, and I need more time to figure them out.

I'm intrigued by the program that fires the electrodes randomly; I think it is developing into my "music" program. We were at an "Irish Festival." (St. Patrick's Day is coming!) There was live entertainment, a singer with drum and electronic instruments as accompaniment, on a big stage with huge speakers broadcasting Irish ballads and drinking songs. The program I was using for speech was behaving weirdly, setting off electronic reverberations instead of transmitting music. This was how my piano had sounded when I first got my CI. The music was not being processed correctly. This sounded like a job for — my music program! I flipped the dial — and, thup-thup — a few seconds later, I was in "music mode." (The speech processor, by the way, makes this "thup-thup" sound as it changes to a new program.) Playing with the volume (slightly down) and the sensitivity (way down), the music literally "came into focus." This was definitely a case of "less is more." The electronic warp pretty much disappeared. I was close enough to read the singer's lips and could understand much of the lyrics. This sounded like music, even though it was unfamiliar to me. I can honestly say that I don't know any Irish drinking songs — yet.

We had dinner out with friends, the noisy restaurant routine again. I'm starting to hit my stride in this situation, plugging in my auxiliary mic.

I don't wear it on myself anymore; I clip it to the tablecloth or just leave it on the table beside me. This seems to have a few advantages over either clipping it to me or somewhere in the middle of the table. I don't hear my own voice too loud this way, so I don't speak too softly. And by keeping it close to me on the table, the wire doesn't end up in the soup.

I've retreated somewhat from my stronger program. It has a fuller sound but I don't necessarily do better with it. After three months, I'm starting to appreciate the rhythm of this CI — try, hear, learn, adjust — over and over again. At three months, I understand it well enough to work patiently with the process. It may not always sound the way I would like, nor do I always hear as well as I would like, but . . . there is no but. It's still a miracle.

DAY 108
MARCH 18

I made my first pay phone call. I can't even remember if I had ever made one before. We were sitting in an airport lounge, waiting for our flight to board with nothing to do but wait. I saw the bank of pay phones with people chatting away. I had always looked at them, wondering what they had so much to talk about. I had effectively removed the idea of ever using a pay phone from my list of things to do. I was painfully aware of the lack of TTY pay phones and had long ago come to terms with the reality of that situation.

The phone bank beckoned. My real concern was that the airline terminal was not quiet and I was wondering if I would be able to hear on the phone with the background noise. I already had a Calling Card, which I had never used, so I was ready. Sure, I was ready, but I had no idea what to *do*! I asked Ira, figuring he was a seasoned pro at this. He told me to dial 1-800-CALLATT, so that I would be hooked up to reliable AT&T, and then listen to the options and follow the directions. That seemed simple enough — IF — and that was a big "if" — I could hear the directions.

As Ira explained this to me, our friends, waiting with us, looked on, following this conversation. We've known them for a long time, and they were well acquainted with my hearing history. From the expressions on their faces, I knew that it had not occurred to them that I had never been able to make pay phone calls before getting my CI. For over 25 years, I may not have been able to make a pay phone call, but I had acquired the knack of reading facial expressions!

Cool Arlene swaggered over to the phone bank. May as well act like the natives when you feel like an alien. I picked up the receiver, making sure that I had chosen a volume-control phone. I pushed the volume-control button to reach a comfortable level, then I punched in 1-800-CALLATT. Actually, it was a little slower than that. First I put on my glasses to see the phone buttons and the letters above the buttons. I'm still such a novice at touch-tone phones, I don't know which letters go with which buttons without looking.

I got the AT&T message, pressed in the numbers of my Calling Card but screwed up the PIN number. The message told me that it didn't recognize what I was punching in. I felt like a beginner, and I must have looked like one too, as I struggled with the phone dial. Start again. 1-800-CALLATT, press in menu numbers, get the right PIN number in, punch in the phone number I was dialing — and . . . YES! It was ringing.

I called my sister and I called my son. "I'm calling you from the airport!" And with that, I was satisfied that I could confidently join the ranks of pay phone users. I noticed that these pay phones were mounted in semi-circular acoustical "booths." When I leaned into a "booth," it muffled the sounds around me and that did help. There was carpeting on the floor, and it wasn't very noisy — certainly not as bad as some other airport locations, so I'm not sure how I would do if I had more noise to contend with. I think I could deal with it, finding a quieter location if need be. I returned to my husband and friends, smiling smugly. Mission accomplished.

There is an irony here, something that those who know me are probably wondering about, so I guess I should "tell all." TTY pay phones do exist, although they are few and far between. As I mentioned, I had pretty much conditioned myself not to expect to find TTY pay phones, so I never bothered to learn how to use them, or took the time to try them on the rare occasion that there was one available. I was not thrilled about this situation, but figured I had other things to worry about. Until. . . .

I was coming home on the Garden State Parkway last spring and I stopped at one of the rest areas. It was late and I wanted to call home to let my family know that I was on my way. There were 40 *volume-control phones* (yes, forty)! There were *no* TTY pay phones. Not one. This was outrageous, but at least I was in a position to do something about it.

On my way home, I drafted a letter, in my head, to the governor. I am a member of the New Jersey Division of the Deaf and Hard of Hearing (DDHH) Advisory Council, an unpaid governor-appointed position. I've traipsed around the state to various meetings fulfilling the responsibilities of this position, driving on state highways that had no phones that I could use. Here I was doing what the governor had appointed me to do, yet the roadway authorities denied me communication access, which was not only a violation of the ADA, but it also put me and others like me in a vulnerable position unnecessarily. When I got home, I typed the letter out, stating the case calmly and honestly. I submitted it to the DDHH. They typed it on DDHH-AC letterhead, I signed it and it was sent to the governor with copies to the commissioners of the highways.

To make a long story short, a few months later, TTY pay phones were installed at all the rest areas on the Garden State Parkway and the New Jersey Turnpike. They still haven't put up enough signs, but all in good time. I feel a little guilty now. I know I should have tried the TTY phones when they were first installed, but that was around the time of my CI surgery, recovery and hookup and I had other things on my mind. It's an ironic swan song, making my debut as a regular pay phone user, just as the TTY pay phones are installed on the highways.

DAY 109
MARCH 19

My Walkman is starting to get a workout. Listening to books on tape is becoming a favorite activity and I look forward to those sessions. It makes my "power walks" much more interesting, and I stay out longer, entranced by the constant flow of words into my head. Listening directly through this recorder is much easier than listening on the car player — no road noise and no distance from the speakers to get in the way. I'm missing very few words, so there is no need to rewind to listen again and therefore no need to hold the player in my hand. It has been relegated to my pocket, with patch cord snaking under my jacket to plug right into my speech processor. No one knows that I am listening to anything, unlike the ubiquitous headphones seen on joggers and other power walkers. Ah — the advantages of being bionic!

The cassette tape version of General Norman Schwarzkopf's memoirs caught my attention in the library, so I decided to tackle it — all four tapes. There is virtually no aspect of my life that hasn't been touched by my hearing problems. And, true to form, General Schwarzkopf's memoirs were not immune. As soon as I heard his voice (he, too, was narrating his own memoirs), it threw me back in time to 1990-1991 and Desert Storm, the Persian Gulf War. I remember watching the Pentagon briefings that he gave to the press. They were captioned, and at that time, I could hear his voice and follow the captions. Those were the only television updates on the war that had captions. CNN's live broadcasts didn't have captioning in those days and anyone relying on captioning was left wondering what was happening when CNN was airing this historic coverage.

I had a particular interest in the details of Desert Storm because, on the suggestion of "Dear Abby," I had written a "Dear Any Serviceperson" letter and sent it to the Army address provided. My letter was answered by a young soldier, Jeff, who was a Huey helicopter technician stationed in the deserts of Saudi Arabia. The news on television was forever changed once I knew an actual person involved in that conflict. As we corresponded, my letters were carefully crafted to inspire courage and strength of spirit. I never mentioned my hearing problems because there was obviously no reason to.

Listening to General Schwarzkopf describing his version of Desert Storm was fascinating because I could match it with Jeff's version, and they meshed. General Schwarzkopf recounted his frustrations trying to eliminate the Scud missile threat, and how carefully he had devised an offensive strategy to minimize casualties. Jeff's letters described the Scud missiles booming overhead as he prepared me for the possibility of his death.

At the end of the war, I wrote to Jeff telling him to call me if he was ever in my area of the country. I didn't anticipate that he would do that anytime soon, but he actually did. He had a stopover at Kennedy Airport on his way back to Fort Bragg, and he called me. I didn't know what to say. I had never mentioned my hearing loss and was finding it very difficult to understand him on the phone. Those were the last few days before I decided to give up using a regular voice phone altogether. I explained my hearing loss and it seemed sort of trivial considering that the person on the other end of the phone was alive and not a casualty of war. They say everything seems trivial after facing a war.

Ira and I eventually met Jeff that summer, visiting Fort Bragg as we made a vacation tour of North Carolina. It was an incredible experience to actually meet the person behind the letters. We had become friends through pen and paper, but now the words literally jumped off the page — a storybook character coming to life! It made me realize how powerful the written word can be, that you could know someone so well without having met them.

We took Jeff out to dinner at what turned out to be a very noisy restaurant. I had come prepared to hear in noise, though. This was the very first time that I was trying an auxiliary microphone with my hearing aid and I was very hesitant about using it. I felt like someone with a limp now needing crutches. It was the "next step" in the downward spiral. When we were seated, with the background music booming, I gave the auxiliary mic to Jeff to put on his collar. He asked, "Can you hear me?" and I smiled, "Yes, I can hear you!" I thought I'd be embarrassed, but I wasn't. This was another of those situations that suddenly seemed trivial in light of the recent war. Here was someone who could have died, so why should I care that it took a microphone and a wire to hear him? I didn't care what it looked like, and I haven't cared ever since.

Those who have seen me use an auxiliary mic with my hearing aid know that it had almost become my trademark. At first, I only used it in noise, but eventually I used it just to hear, period. It brought in every last bit of usable sound enabling me to lipread. I've often been asked if I felt uneasy about holding it up to people's faces "interview-style." "No," I would always reply. I didn't have a problem with it, and if other people did, that was their problem. Thinking back on how and when I made my auxiliary mic debut, even a question like that seemed petty and naive.

The auxiliary mic for my CI is smaller than the one for my hearing aid, and I only use it when there is a lot of background noise. As I become more accustomed to listening in noise, I'm finding that I'm using it less and I've only held it up "interview-style" once. I wouldn't hesitate a moment to do that again if I had to. There's nothing quite like being able to say, "Yes, I can hear you."

DAY 121
MARCH 22

I'm starting to develop a relationship with my brain, appreciating its power over my hearing. The key to all this "it will keep getting better" talk, is predicated on the brain learning how to hear with this implant, and I keep witnessing this learning process. I am really in awe, and humbled. I recall somewhere in a junior high school science class being told that humans only use about 10% of the capacity of the brain. This implant is definitely forcing mine into new territory. Yes, I'll explain.

About two weeks ago, I turned on my car's CD player and tuned into the Chopin piano music I had recently bought. I didn't have the case for this CD, with its table of contents, so I didn't know what, specifically, I was listening to. All I could tell was that it did sound like Chopin piano music. About a week or so ago, I listened again, and I could tell that the first piece was the "Raindrop Prelude," something I had played — oh, about 35 years ago. It has a distinctive bass line that is supposed to sound like raindrops. I strained to hear the melody line, but couldn't get it. Yesterday, I tuned into the same piece and the melody jumped out at me. Goodness — what happened? The only conclusion is that my brain did it; somehow, it got better at distinguishing the individual sounds of the music.

That's one example. Now consider this one. When I put on my speech processor in the morning, my husband invariably has the radio turned to the morning news. For years, I hated the sound of that radio through my hearing aid because it was just raucous noise. It's a 28-year-old

Sony model with genuine wood trim — a real relic, but it works. I would always turn it off as soon as my husband left the room.

I must have gotten into the habit because I have still been turning it off in the morning, even now. I can't really understand it from across the room, and I had no desire to bother with it. Now that I am realizing that my brain can be trained, I thought I'd give this radio a chance. I had been able to hear some of it up close, but not from across the room. I figured I'd let my brain listen for a while, just to let it get used to the sound. I puttered around the room, making the bed, hanging up clothes, not really paying attention to the radio. After a few minutes, I heard a "1-800" phone number announced. Hmmm, was my brain taking the bait? Seemed so. I kept puttering — and as I kept listening, I started to get some words. First a woman announcer, then a male. I didn't want to stress myself out trying to catch every word; it wasn't that important. I was just curious about the idea of letting my brain get used to different sounds, even raucous radio sounds from a distance. I'm finding that it does sometimes take a little time to get adjusted to some hearing environments and sounds.

Today I was at a choral concert. My friend, Susan, was singing and she invited me to come. Susan is one of the "Sewing Lady" volunteers, and she also shares my love of music. I declined the invitation to her last concert, in December, because I didn't think I could enjoy a concert so soon after my hookup. But this time, I decided to give it a try. I sat up front, figuring that closer would be better. There was no amplification system in use. The program was all jazz, with a jazz combo playing — drums, bass, sax, piano, trombone — nothing electronic.

It took the entire first song to tune into it. I tried using each of my three programs with and without the auxiliary mic. My headpiece microphone worked better, and the strong flat program worked best, with the sensitivity turned down, but not all the way. My "music program" didn't sound as good as the flat program. I'm still learning, that's for sure. I sat and listened. By tuning in the volume and the sensitivity, I got it to sound as natural as I could. The sensitivity adjustment was important — too low, and it wouldn't pick up enough sound — too high, and it would take on an electronic "warp."

First of all, it sounded like music. That is *not* a given. It could have sounded like electronic mush. I could identify it as choral music. The percussion sounded the truest. The piano wasn't bad. I could hear the soloists. I decided to leave the settings and just listen, again giving my brain a chance to absorb the sound.

I can say that this is a good approach, not only for music or clock radios across the room. It is good to give everything a chance and not declare it too hard to hear, or not natural enough. I really think that it all needs a chance, and my brain deserves the chance to keep learning. That is why I say that I am developing a relationship with my brain. I've seen it in action, and I sure wish I had some control over this process. I feel like Sherlock Holmes giving the "scent" to the bloodhounds. Okay, brain, here's some raw sound, learn to live with it, and make it sound the way it should.

For the same reason, I continue to listen to books on tape. It's a dangerous pursuit because I get hooked on them and can't seem to tear myself away. In addition to General Schwarzkopf, Russell Baker, Alan Dershowitz and several others, I just completed listening to Helen Hayes narrating her life story, *In Three Acts*. She was lovely to listen to. Obviously, her diction is impeccable, a delight to hear. I found that after listening to her for three hours, I started to talk like her. (I wish!) She enunciates her consonants so beautifully and so precisely. It reminded me how much difference it makes in my own speech to be able to hear myself again.

Although I had retained excellent speech despite my hearing loss, I know that I am enunciating much more precisely now. I can hear it. I'm also realizing that some of my friends, who have profound hearing losses, don't enunciate as well as I thought they did. I'm actually having more trouble understanding them now that I can hear them than I did when I was relying mostly on lipreading. I was trying to figure out why this should be, and it was fairly obvious. Anyone who has had speech therapy is trained to make the proper lip movements. But the tongue and mouth movements that aren't seen on the lips are more difficult to reproduce and are often less precise. So for someone who is relying mostly on lipreading to understand, no problem. But for someone who is relying on the sounds, it's more difficult.

And the last little tidbit is that the new stronger flat program, the one that I had been shying away from, is now winning. I've had it almost two weeks, and it's the one that I like to listen to the audio book tapes with. I seem to prefer it to the weaker program that had been my favorite just two weeks ago. Don't ask me how or why this happens. Ask my brain — it seems to have a mind of its own.

DAY 124
APRIL 3

I finally got my chance to fly solo with my CI, something that had been on my mind to do for some time. No, I did not actually fly the plane although with all the planning and preparation, I might just as well have.

I had only flown by myself twice before, both times to Self Help for Hard of Hearing People (SHHH) conventions. It was not an experience I would recommend to people without hearing. It was always so emotionally and physically taxing. I felt like an animal on the prowl, senses on "high alert" with eyes scanning the scenery. Missing announcements was my greatest fear, aside from being run over by beeping airport trams. Asking people what the announcements were saying was out of the question because my hearing was too poor even to know that there *were* announcements. And asking for assistance was difficult because I wasn't sure that I would understand the reply. Something as simple as being asked my beverage choices on the plane could be a source of confusion and embarrassment, especially if a flight attendant asked me something when I wasn't looking her way. The constant fear of not knowing what was going on was intensely stressful and I hated it.

Now, with my CI, I was ready for my solo flight. I had already flown a few times since getting my CI, accompanied by Ira, so I knew what to expect. Old habits and fears die hard, though. When I had no hearing, planning, at least for known contingencies, was essential. This habit carried over with my CI because I couldn't be sure how much I would hear in every circumstance. I had done my homework. I was ready.

I pulled my car into the off-site parking facility at Newark Airport. Although the long-term parking lots are less expensive, there is no assurance that your car will still be there when you return from your trip. Even though publicity for the airport claims their track record is improving, we always park at a private parking facility right outside the airport. I knew that I wouldn't have to go into the office when dropping off my car, and that the outside attendants would ask me when I was returning and on what flight. I can't tell you how many questions I actually heard and what I understood because of my "preparation." I do know that I hopped aboard the shuttle bus without my blood pressure rising.

Once in the airline terminal, I checked in right away even though I wasn't checking any baggage. I knew that they now require photo ID, so I had that ready. I also expected them to ask me if my luggage had been out of my sight, and some other security questions. I was fine with all this. I was wearing my auxiliary microphone because I knew I would be moving in and out of noisy areas, and the auxiliary mic would serve me best in these varying environments.

Safely checked in, I headed for the gate, which meant that I had to pass through the security scanners. Other airports have an area where you can walk around them, but not Newark. I knew I would set off the alarms. I have learned that it is probably the external speech processor which sets them off, so the choice is between taking the speech processor off or leaving it on and being patted down. My choice is to be patted down because I would rather not be left without hearing, even for a few moments, especially in a security situation. Who knows what sort of questions they might ask me?

I also knew that if I set my carry-on luggage and handbag on the conveyor belt, they would go through but I would not be there to retrieve them right away once I had set off the alarms. I anticipated this, so when the alarms did go off, I told the security people to retrieve my bags for me. Once they had set them aside, I told them that I had a medical device and would have to be patted down. They usually get a woman to do that and it takes only a few seconds. I picked up my bags and was on my way. It's taking me more time to describe this whole security encounter than it actually takes to go through it.

At the gate, I was early. I knew Ira was supposed to be picking me up from the airport when I landed; I was joining him at a convention in Orlando. So far everything was right on schedule. I passed a bank of pay phones. "Ah," they beckoned, "you know how to use us now. Real people phone their family to make sure that they know you are on the way." I took the hint.

I picked a phone with volume control in an area that was carpeted. This would muffle some of the background noise. Unfortunately, there was a constant barrage of announcements, so it was not the "quiet location" I had hoped for. I'm glad this wasn't my first phone call because it was a more difficult hearing environment than when I had tried a pay phone a few weeks before. I got out my calling card, pushed the numbers, and I was in! I got the hotel Ira was staying in, asked for the extension, got voice mail options, left a message saying that everything was going according to schedule, then hung up. I wanted to tell everyone nearby that I had just made my first "real" pay phone call! The other calls didn't count because they were practice. But nobody would have cared. I did just what everyone else does in an airport. But that's all I wanted, really — to be like everyone else.

I took a seat by the departure gate. I knew I would be able to hear the flight announcements, but that I might not be able to understand them. I heard the first announcement and saw people getting up to board the plane. I asked the woman sitting next to me if they were calling seat numbers yet. "No," she said. That question and answer was a triumph in itself. I had no doubt this time that I would be able to hear the person next to me, so my blood pressure stayed put, and this animal did not have to go on "high alert." I watched the attendant at the gate, and after a few minutes, I heard "Row 25 and above" being called to board the plane. That was me! I heard the announcement, maybe I saw her announce it, too. Whatever — I got up, and I was on my way!

There's no need to describe the flight; it was uneventful. I could hear some of the announcements over the loudspeaker. I knew when the flight attendant was talking to me, and beverage and snack preferences were no problem. A diet Pepsi and peanuts — with no hearing, making those choices correctly without embarrassment would have been a triumph. With my CI — trivial.

We touched down on time. The Eagle had landed. I gathered my belongings, headed up the aisle, and walked calmly through the exit ramp. Ira was waiting for me as I set foot in the terminal. One small step for me and my CI, one huge leap for my quality of life.

DAY 126
APRIL 5

My first solo flight to Orlando delivered me to one of Ira's business conventions. I have gone to this particular convention many times before and with each successive year, it presented new challenges as my hearing went from bad to worse to none. I doubt that anyone knew how hard I was working to function, while trying to look as if I wasn't working very hard at all. As a "spouse," I was lucky; at least I didn't have to conduct any business. All I had to do was look and sound charming and intelligent. Lest that task be too easy, somewhere it had been decreed that I would have to do this without hearing. I'm sure this builds character, but I can't say I would have chosen this method. I often felt as if I was on "Beat the Clock," the '50's game show. Go in there and do what everyone else is doing, but do it standing on one foot with one hand tied behind your back.

There was no doubt in my mind that my CI was going to make a *big* difference in how I would function this time. I might even have fun, a word that wasn't even in my vocabulary before. The name of the game had always been "function," not "fun."

It started with a "spouse breakfast." Conventions are usually geared to "business breakfasts" so they have to do something with the spouses. As expected, I had to "fly solo" right away. Ira had meetings. I met some women coming to breakfast and started chatting with them. BIG DIF-FERENCE NUMBER 1! I had never casually chatted with anyone. There were large round tables and I sat down and joined the conversation with some other women. BIG DIFFERENCE NUMBER 2! I had never done *that* before either. I was never able to talk with more than one person at a time.

I was really starting to like breakfast even though it was only bagels and juice. I've skipped them in the past simply because I didn't want to deal with talking to people. Being on my own in unfamiliar territory was usually taxing enough. I'd also had my fill of embarrassing episodes, where I couldn't figure out what was going on or what to do. I even developed my own vocabulary for those situations: being "beaten up."

I wasn't surprised about breezing through breakfast with my CI, but I did savor the experience. Nice not to start the day being "beaten up." No waitresses asking me for my room number when I thought they were offering me more coffee, or similar indignities. Calm. Happy. Pleasant. Yes, "breakfast with my CI" was fun.

Being in a hotel had always posed a problem for me because I had to use a TTY, making it virtually impossible for other people to call my room. I had always reconciled myself to just letting the chips fall, not going to great lengths to try to open telephone communications with other people at the convention. For years, I had also been afraid to pick up a ringing phone. What would I say? It was all too complicated. I had watched with wonder as Ira called for information, messages, dinner arrangements, parking — all with such ease. I had always looked on, resigned to the reality that hotel phones were for other people, not for me. Oh sure, I had always requested TTY service in my room and at the front desk, and gotten it. But it was never easy, it didn't always work, and I didn't think many people would be willing to maneuver through this obstacle course to call me, even if they knew how. Now that I could use a regular voice phone, I was reachable! BIG DIFFERENCE NUMBER 3! And, lo and behold, someone did phone me to say they would be late meeting me in the lobby. I answered the phone, and I heard them.

It was also apparent that I wasn't going to have to dig into my bag of tricks, or use all my wiles to "do" this convention. My brain was starting to talk to me again. "When am I going to have to *think*, Arlene?" I felt like a baseball player who had practiced for years with a donut on his bat and had finally taken off the extra weight. This was all too easy. Is this what everyone else usually experiences? No wonder they always looked as if they were having fun!

The next test was the dinner party, beginning with cocktails. These noisy events had always been my biggest challenge: how to sound charming and intelligent when I couldn't hear a thing. Just as Donald Trump can tell you about "the art of the deal," I can tell you about the art of the manipulated conversation. I don't think I ever consciously figured out how to do this; it was a sink or swim situation, usually based on the premise that if you talk, you don't have to listen. But if you talk too much, you won't be charming, so you have to engage the other person in conversation by asking questions where it matters not at all what the answers are. This guaranteed that I would always know the topic of conversation and it also appeared as if I was interested in the answer. I *was* interested in what other people had to say, but I could never afford myself that luxury. My brain was always in overdrive — always — because not only did it need to have command of the current events of the day and the business trends of the moment, remembering appropriate humorous anecdotes and other relevant tidbits, it also had to lipread the responses with little or no sound. I'm sure that people had no idea what it meant not to be able to hear or what hard work it was.

At this dinner party, I learned something new. Even I never realized how hard I had been working just to stay in a "small talk" conversation at a dinner party. As I stood there, conversing with people I knew from previous conventions, I didn't have to work. I was expecting my brain to start whizzing and whirring. It never happened. It didn't need to — I could hear the people I was talking to. I had fully expected that it would all be much easier, but I never expected to be shocked to learn just how much. I am still shocked.

And that's pretty much how the convention went. My brain kept nudging me, "When am I going to have to *think*, Arlene?" Sorry, brain, just keep adjusting to the CI. I can handle this with my hearing.

DAY 131
APRIL 10

Orlando is the home of Disney World. The last time Ira and I visited was when their new MGM Studios theme park opened several years ago. What a disaster that was!

Silly me, I had thought since I had used the infrared system at a few EPCOT attractions many years before, MGM would at least have that available. With the increased prevalence of closed captioning on television, I assumed they would have that as well. On that visit, MGM was a sea of movie screens, television sets, and wheelchair ramps, with absolutely no provision made for deaf and hard of hearing people. Oh, I shouldn't say that. They did have a TTY telephone available at their Guest Relations center. Why they thought that people in wheelchairs came to see the attractions, yet deaf and hard of hearing people only came to Disney World to make phone calls was beyond me.

I was so upset at the time that I complained vehemently by letter to the management. They placated me by refunding my admission price, I guess figuring that would keep me quiet. Comparing notes with others, I was not the only one upset by the lack of assistive devices for deaf and hard of hearing people. Evidently, a lawsuit by the family of a deaf child, and the eager attendees of the SHHH convention in Orlando in 1996 made Disney finally decide to face up to its ADA responsibilities.

If I sound particularly bitter, it's because I also recall, many years ago, being given what were supposed to have been the scripts of the attractions. One of the "scripts" said that I would be watching a funny movie where the characters would be having a very humorous conversation. It never bothered to tell me what the characters were saying or what was so funny. This from the geniuses who were developing state-of-the-art entertainment! I remember sitting there not understanding a thing while the entire audience was convulsed with laughter. I complained by letter then too and got a "we'll refer this to the appropriate people" response, which amounted to no response.

So with that as background, I again ventured into MGM Studios the first day and EPCOT the next, this time armed with my CI and the knowledge that Disney had made improvements in accessibility. I knew that they had installed more infrared systems, as well as closed captioning (CC) systems for some attractions and television screens. I headed straight to Guest Relations for the needed equipment and instructions. A smiling Mouseketeer, *sans* ears, provided me with an infrared receiver that could accommodate my CI patch cord, and also a tv clicker to turn on any televisions that were marked with a "CC" symbol. I was instructed to tell the attendants at the attractions with the "Reflective Captioning" that I needed to use this service. Now to actually try out these gizmos. I had learned from bitter experience that even having good intentions doesn't guarantee that the equipment will work.

THE TV CLICKER   After two days of walking around the theme parks looking for "CC" tv screens to click on, I found that nothing worked — except for one tv that was *not* marked. This was an individual screen at the "Tower of Terror" with Rod Serling talking. It had no CC marking, but responded with captions to the zap of the clicker — sort of like Marcel Marceau saying "No" in Mel Brooks' film, *Silent Movie* — the mute mime being the only one to talk in the entire film.

Why none of the other tv screens responded to my clicker is yet unknown and, of course, I didn't have time to try each and every screen in the park. It was most likely a battery problem. What annoyed me was that they would go to such lengths to *hide* the captioning. Most attractions with tv screens had a dozen or more in one location. Would it really have destroyed their esthetics to permanently caption a few of them? There is no doubt that many people who would have welcomed the captioning either didn't know about this clicker system or didn't bother to get one. I also would have welcomed one less thing to carry around.

THE INFRARED SYSTEM   The guide maps showed which attractions had infrared systems, but it was still difficult to determine exactly where they were working. In some attractions, the waiting area had infrared. In others, only the main entertainment area did. So I kept trying. I wasn't disgruntled though. (Years of being "beaten up" had taught me patience and gratitude.) This was already a big improvement over my previous visits.

That said, it was still a hit or miss experience. The "Beauty and the Beast" show was in a very open, canopied arena, where the infrared signal was so weak and static-y that it was useless. Weren't these imagineers aware that too much light can kill an infrared signal? Was there perhaps a section of the audience where it worked best? I don't know. There were no signs, and I wondered if they had ever tested the system.

Ira and I had a better experience at another MGM attraction, "SuperStar Television," where they cast some audience members for the show. Most of the casting was done in the waiting area, where there was no infrared so I couldn't follow everything. Once inside, though, the emcee's hand-held mic was working clear as a bell with the infrared. She asked, "Is there anyone in the audience celebrating an anniversary?" and I shot my hand up. "How many years?" she continued. "Twenty-eight," I replied. With that, Ira and I were ushered backstage for the episode that required a married couple. Ira immediately asked me, "Why did you raise your hand?" I told him, "Because I heard the question!"

Let me explain this. I have never heard anything like this so clearly. This was "Gold" hearing. I heard it and the meaning went straight to my brain which responded instantly. It was almost as if it was waiting 27 years to answer a question like that. Perhaps my brain hasn't learned yet that it doesn't *have* to respond immediately to everything it hears and understands, but I guess that will come with time. The irony was that there was no infrared transmitter backstage, so I couldn't understand much of the show.

In EPCOT, they gave me an infrared receiver that had channels. This receiver worked well in "The American Adventure" pavilion, which tells the history of the United States using a multi-media show with computer-animated figures. I figured out what the channels were for when Benjamin Franklin started speaking Spanish to Mark Twain. Flipped the channel — German. Flipped again — French. This was so cool! I finally found English. I remember going to this pavilion years ago without the infrared system and not understanding anything. As real as computer-animated figures look, they cannot be lipread. (That holds true for Muppets as well.)

THE REFLECTIVE CAPTIONING SYSTEM   Several attractions had "Reflective Captioning," and these locations were indicated on the guide map. With this system, the captions are displayed backwards at the rear of the hall and when you position a portable transparent screen to see the reflection of the captions, you can read them in front of you. This is like putting ECNALUBMA on the front of an ambulance so that you can read it correctly from your car's rear-view mirror. The only problem with the system was that you had to notify the attendant as people were filing into the auditorium, and they had to set you up in the few moments before the shows. This didn't leave much time to get settled and seated properly. I was pleased with the way the system worked, though, and happy I didn't have to shlep around special equipment.

So, yes — I had a better time at Disney World this time around. I only went to EPCOT and MGM, so I don't know about the other theme parks, but EPCOT was the clear winner here. Most of the attractions there had infrared, with many of them also equipped with the reflective captioning. I actually had fun, and didn't feel like an outsider, as I had in the past. It was far from perfect, but definitely a worthy effort.

DAY 135
APRIL 14

I attended a meeting last week and as soon as it began, I knew that I was doing "better." I was hearing at a distance "better" and that meant that it was approaching more "normal" hearing.

How much better was I doing? I didn't even have to glance at the captioning. I got all the speech by hearing and watching the speakers. The "better" part became apparent when I realized that I could even follow some of the speakers when I wasn't looking at them. That was eerie and I'm not totally comfortable with it yet, but it was interesting to see my progress, measured by my ability to function at a meeting I had been to before.

Why this progress, this very noticeable progress? I keep thinking about it. Probably, my hearing would get better over time with just the routine of daily life providing the practice of listening to speech. But I am convinced that listening to the audio books on tape has also made a difference.

Listening to the audio books is something like perfecting a tennis stroke; it's strengthening, conditioning and coordinating the paths to the brain. It's not so different from hitting a tennis ball against a wall over and over again, something I did a millennium ago, while perfecting a two-handed backhand to overcome a weak forearm. Again and again, I banged that ball until my backhand became my best shot.

My hearing in noise has also improved, and I'm wondering if listening to the tapes has helped that as well, training my brain to pull out those speech sounds. I am fortunate not to have to follow the written text when I listen, so I can play my tapes anywhere. There is no such thing as "down time" for me anymore, those huge expanses of time when I was driving or walking, when there was absolutely nothing to do but think. All that time can now be filled if I want to. I can listen to tapes in the car or with my Walkman. With the Walkman, I'm plugged in directly, so there is no background noise at all. But in the car, there's plenty of road noise — and the faster, the noisier. The sound quality of my tape player is much better without high-speed road noise distractions, so I don't mind getting stuck in traffic anymore!

I have been resisting the temptation to discuss the tapes I have been listening to. Non-fiction is the order of the day not only because it interests me more, but it is easier to listen to than fiction, no dramatizations and background music, just straight text. My head is being loaded with ideas and information. I'm not sure where I'm going to store it all! For someone who was raised with the notion that idle time is sin, this new-found use of previously unusable time presents mind-boggling opportunities. I've already fought through the Civil War, discovering that everything I had learned in school had been whitewashed, literally. I've combed through the lives of some famous people, learning that they were human, the secret of their success being hard work, a belief in themselves, and a little bit of luck. Russell Baker, Norman Schwartzkopf, Helen Hayes, Leonard Nimoy, Neil Simon, Alan Dershowitz — I'm starting to lose track as my brain is being crammed full.

I am definitely getting better at this. Using the Walkman, most of my hearing is in that "Gold" range, hearing it and understanding it. Not all, though. For more difficult tapes, like the one about the Civil War, I got all the words but had to rewind sometimes to get the meaning — Silver hearing. Facts were flowing too fast and furiously.

In the car, it is still difficult, but that, too, is better. I brought that Civil War tape with me, figuring that I'd never be able to understand it — they spoke so fast — but I did. From that I knew that this tape-listening must be accelerating whatever progress I am destined to make. It was not a fluke that I performed significantly better at the meeting I had just attended.

I also remember where I was when listening to these tapes — where in my neighborhood I was walking when Helen Hayes made her acting debut, where I was driving when Neil Simon's wife died, and what stretch of the Garden State Parkway I was on when General Schwartzkopf was commanding the Gulf War. Mother Nature may have some useful purpose for this behavioral quirk although I have yet to fathom what it is.

DAY 143
APRIL 22

I'm starting to forget what it was like not to hear. No, I shouldn't really say that. I don't hear every night when I take off my speech processor. I thought I'd be in a panic of sorts, having to go from hearing all day to silence. For some reason, that doesn't seem to bother me. When I had my hearing aid, I wasn't hearing much anyway, so taking off the hearing aid at night was almost a relief. It's not that way with the speech processor. It's just another fact of life: make the usual preparations to go to sleep and then take off the speech processor — just one more thing to do. One day, I guess I'll be taking out my teeth too.

I really am starting to forget what it was like not to hear though. I imagine myself in a ship, going further and further away from that shore of deafness and it is getting more distant each day. Over four months now, enough time to be convinced that yes, this is now my hearing, not some hope or dream. For four months, I haven't experienced any loss in hearing, and subtly, I'm starting to realize that. I haven't gone four months without losing hearing in almost thirty years.

These past four months, I've been using only a voice phone, no Relay, no TTY's. Some calls are easier than others, but not once was I in such trouble that I thought of using Relay. I still have my TTY equipment out and ready to use, but I've only used my amplified telephones. That feature is still helpful for me, allowing me to adjust the volume to suit my needs.

I hadn't realized how accustomed I had become to the speed of voice telephone communications until just the other day. I wanted to place a phone order to Lands' End, the mail order company. Before my CI, I always used to dial their TTY number and place my order TTY to TTY, rather than use Relay. That way I could type my credit card number, name and address. It was a very efficient way to place a phone order, or so I thought. With my CI, I figured that calling TTY to TTY would still be an efficient way to place a mail order, until I actually tried it again.

Using a TTY again felt a little strange, but I dialed the number. The sales person typed back, so s-l-o-w-l-y, "Hello. How may I help you?" "Okay," I thought, "it's sort of slow, but it always worked so well for me." So I typed back that I wanted to place an order. The sales person typed back, so s-l-o-w-l-y, saying she needed the number on the back of the catalogue. At that point, I realized that I didn't want to sit there forever typing out this order, and she still had to ask me about colors and quantities and size and anything else to order — oh, so s-l-o-w-l-y. So I quickly typed back "have to go, sorry" — and I hung up. I then dialed the voice number, got another sales person, told her the catalogue information, size, color, quantity and that was all I was ordering. That took about a minute. I had been transformed. Life had sped up for me and I hadn't even noticed. I no longer had the patience to do what I previously thought was terrific.

While I know that I'm getting better at hearing in noise, it's still not so good if the background noise is music. The sounds seem to get merged. Just the other day I ran into friends in a store where there was background music playing, and I couldn't understand them — at all. I didn't panic. I knew that if I pulled out my auxiliary mic, I'd be fine. When I *know* that I'm going to be in noise, then it's easy. I plug in my auxiliary mic ahead of time. But getting caught unexpectedly in noise, that's my weakness. Alas, even Superman had his Kryptonite!

As I continue to listen to books on audio tape, I'm still amazed that I can understand so well. I don't know how many times I've mentioned this, but I'll say it again: if anyone had told me a mere five months ago that I would be able to listen to books on tape, I would have said it was too preposterous to contemplate. I recall, on the eve of my CI, wondering if some of the wonderful success stories I had been hearing about could possibly happen to me. I couldn't even imagine it, and now, I'm living it.

I'm concerned that I'm painting too glowing a picture about my CI progress, that people might get the idea that this CI gives me normal hearing. At the same time, I also hesitate to "complain" because it is making such a difference in my life. Even with its quirks, it is nothing short of miraculous. Do you suppose the Israelites complained about mud in their sandals when they crossed the Red Sea? Same principle. So miracle, yes — perfect, no.

DAY 147
APRIL 26

I attended a meeting last week of the New Jersey Division of the Deaf and Hard of Hearing Advisory Council. These are quarterly meetings, and since I had missed the last one, this was the first time I had attended since getting my CI. I don't know sign language, so all my communication has always relied on my lipreading skills and my residual hearing. I always managed to do all right communicating with this group, where there were many deaf and hard of hearing people in attendance. Many of them know sign language, and they usually sign as they speak. The signing never helped me, but it did slow down their speech, which made it easier for me to lipread.

I was curious how this meeting would go with my CI. I had attended smaller meetings, and had functioned very well, able to hear just about everyone around a table of 12 to 15 people. There were twice as many people here, and the room was much larger. Realtime captioning was provided as well as interpreters and an infrared listening system. I had already decided not to use the infrared because I was concerned about hearing my own voice accurately. I usually spoke quite a bit at these meetings, and it was important for me to be able to modulate the volume level of my voice. If I used the infrared system, I would only hear my voice if I spoke directly into a microphone. I figured that with my past successes at the smaller meetings, I would be able to understand those around me, and I could glance at the captioning for anything I missed.

Just describing this planning process is reminder enough that the CI is not normal hearing, especially where distance is concerned. I am still a novice at this, so I decided to stay calm and just roll with the punches.

Many of the people who attend this meeting have a profound hearing loss. Before getting my CI, I had been able to detect the nasal quality of their voices that usually accompanies a profound hearing loss. Their lip movements were always "normal," so I never had much trouble understanding them. I arrived early enough to be able to chat with some of my friends. I was all geared up with my auxiliary microphone because I knew it would be a noisy environment. As I listened, I started to realize that I was having difficulty understanding the people who had a profound hearing loss. I still heard that nasal quality with my CI, but now I was noticing that consonants were distorted or missing.

People had told me that my lipreading skills might diminish over time, through lack of use. At first I thought that was why I was having such trouble. It made sense that if they were not enunciating the consonant sounds, then my lipreading skills should take over. If I was not understanding as well as I used to, then it must be my lipreading skills that were not as sharp as before. Nice theory, but it bothered me. I gave it a lot of thought and concluded that this was not about my lipreading skills.

Before getting my CI, when I heard people who had "deaf speech," I never realized that they were not enunciating their consonants distinctly. I couldn't hear consonants, so I thought that the difference in their speech compared to that of hearing people was just the nasality. My husband had always told me that he had trouble understanding this type of speech, but I never understood why. It seemed normal to me, just the tone was a little different.

With my pre-CI residual hearing, and the visual cues, my brain was getting the words, and the words had consonants, even if I wasn't hearing them. My perception — what was reaching my brain — was complete words. Residual hearing + visual cues = real words. My brain had been filling in the consonants, and if my brain said that there were consonants, who was I to argue?

Now that I can actually hear the consonants, things are subtly changing. When I first heard that *Peter and the Wolf* tape, where the

narrator talks about the wolf coming out of the "for-e-S-T," I remember
my brain doing a doubletake, "WHOA, what was that sound? E-S-T? I
haven't heard that in a long time. Sounds great! If you're going to be giving them to me now, I guess I won't have to imagine them anymore!" Yes,
that is what my CI can deliver — consonants. After four months, my brain
has evidently stopped supplying the missing information. For regular
spoken English, it doesn't need to anymore.

Consider, too, that there was always more to lipreading than
watching lips. Residual hearing was very important, even scant fragments
of sound. When I was using my residual hearing, my brain was learning how
to understand English without the sounds it was no longer being supplied
with. That's why someone who has lost his hearing gradually can understand
a lot more with residual hearing than someone who loses the same amount
of hearing suddenly. The brain has been slowly trained not to need all the
speech sounds. I remember taking a hearing test several years ago. I had to
guess every single word on the list, and I got 80%. If I had been instructed
not to guess, I would have gotten zero. My brain had effectively learned a
slightly different language based on the sound it was being supplied with, and
if my hearing hadn't constantly kept getting worse, I might have gotten very
good at it.

Back at the meeting, the tip-off to this theory was when one of my
friends said that something was "cloh to" his house. I didn't understand, so
I asked him to repeat. There had been no "s" sound in "close" so it came out
"cloh" and my brain didn't process that, even with the visual cue. All that
audio tape listening has also been teaching my brain to automatically rely
on what it hears. This is not the same as losing the ability to lipread. It means
there has been a communication shift from visual to aural.

Analyzing this further, I noticed that, in the speech of my deaf and
hard of hearing friends, along with the "s" sound, the "ch" and "sh" sounds
were missing, and a crisp "t" sound too. I had never noticed this because
before getting my CI, I couldn't hear those sounds either. Being able to hear
my own speech now, I know that I am moving my own tongue differently,
without consciously doing so. The very tip of my tongue, and the exact
placement behind my front teeth is far more precise than it had been. I can
easily tell now how that "s" or "t" sound can become dulled to almost a

"d" sound, or lost entirely if it isn't heard. I guess that's how it's intended to be — hear and imitate. And I also hear a resonance in my voice that I couldn't detect before. People have told me that when I remove the head mic of my CI, to demonstrate what it looks like, my voice changes. I find that incredible that even a brief moment without hearing affects the sound of my voice. This revelation gives me added perspective when conversing with my friends, a deeper understanding of the impact of hearing on speech. And I find myself wishing I could share this precious gift of hearing with them.

DAY 148
APRIL 27

With the arrival of spring, I just experienced my first CI-enhanced baseball game. Ira, being from "da Bronx," is a dyed-in-the-wool Yankee fan. My passion for the game is not as intense as his, but enthusiasm for the Yankees does run in my family. My grandparents' apartment was in the Bronx, and I recall being able to see Yankee Stadium from the roof. There was always someone up there with a radio, tuned to the game, and I remember the sound of those broadcasts — the roar of the crowd, and the "holy cow!'s" of the announcers. My father took me to a game when I was six, and I remember him trying to convince me that watching the Yankees win 1-0 with Whitey Ford pitching was something to get excited about. That may explain my current "enthusiasm."

We've gone to quite a few games over the years. (I'm a good sport.) With my hearing aid and sensitivity to noise, it always presented a challenge. The noise in a stadium filled with beer-drinking, cheering fans is sporadic. Synchronized with the action on the field, the crowd can instantly erupt into an ear-splitting blast and then fall quiet again. I wasn't that much of a fan, but I did enjoy the peanuts and Cracker Jacks, and the opportunity to chat with my friends. I would use my auxiliary microphone with my hearing aid to field whatever speech sounds I could, and I would lipread the rest. When things got really noisy, though, I had to shut everything down. I just couldn't stand the noise with my hearing aid. Another problem was hearing the national anthem. I couldn't. Sometimes I'd follow the lyrics by watching people's mouths, but it was usually a lost cause.

You can imagine my curiosity about hearing my first baseball game with my CI. I knew I was going to do better; it's hard to imagine doing worse. Anything would be an improvement over watching a baseball game like a silent movie.

Dressing for a Yankee game required a little preparation — no ostentatious jewelry. I settled on my little sterling silver whistle, something I realized I hadn't worn since getting my CI. This was understated elegance because it was a Cartier whistle, found in one of the antique flea markets in the city. When we first bought it, Ira said to try it and see if it worked. I blew it with all my might, and instantly produced grotesque pained expressions on the faces of everyone around me. I heard nothing, even with my hearing aid. This was a bizarre little trick, being able to elicit such intense reactions from people without being affected by it myself.

Naturally, as I put on my whistle, I was curious to hear it with my CI. So I popped it in my mouth and blew. Yes — loud and high-pitched! Just the sort of sounds I couldn't hear before. But it wasn't painful. When the comfort and volume levels are adjusted at the mapping sessions, the maximum loudness is set, so I am rarely bothered by very loud sounds. Ahhh, the best of both worlds. I could hear it, but the sound didn't bother me. The advantages of being bionic!

At Yankee Stadium, it was noisy, but never too noisy. I put on my auxiliary mic so that I could hear my friend sitting next to me better. I never had to shut anything down, even during doubles, triples and home runs. And when the "noise meter" urged every fan in the stadium to cheer his loudest, it didn't bother me a bit. Of course, that was my cue to take out my whistle and blow it to my heart's content! No one winced. One only wonders how loud it was in that stadium at the time I was probably the only one there who didn't have to worry about damaging the nerve endings in my cochlea. Mine are already defunct.

How was the Star Spangled Banner? It was a rare opportunity — Robert Merrill was there in person, singing it in front of a microphone. (I have no idea how old he is, but he was singing the national anthem back when Whitey Ford was pitching.) Being broadcast into this cavernous stadium, the sound was not being picked up accurately by my CI. It was mostly echoes and I couldn't really hear his voice as music. I'll just have to be content with my memories of Robert Merrill singing the national anthem. It turns out that CI's are just like baseball — you win some and you lose some.

DAY 165
MAY 14

I am still trying out my new wings in new ways. I had an opportunity to join Ira on a business trip to Chicago, and I jumped at the chance. I don't think I would have if I still couldn't hear. Not being able to hear was stressful enough so I didn't need to look for more. But with five months of CI experience, I had so many things I wanted to see and do, hearing didn't even enter the picture, at least not as something that would hold me back.

Once we were in Chicago, Challenge Number One had me running ahead to check into the hotel while Ira registered for his conference. (No wasted moments are allowed in this family.) I really wanted to do this task "*sans* auxiliary mic," so I turned my sensitivity setting down and proceeded to the lobby counter. I could barely hear the desk clerk. I hadn't realized that directly behind me, the lobby also functioned as an elaborate piano lounge, with the piano going full blast. Background music — that's my weakness. I muddled through, getting my keys, messages, and all the other details, as a hard of hearing person would. No panic, no sinking feelings of "what do I do now?," no despair. I wasn't doing very well, but I knew I could pull out my auxiliary mic if I wanted to. But I didn't want to. I had enough lipreading ability and coping skills to manage. My blood pressure didn't rise as it would have before getting my CI. I was sort of playing with the situation, seeing what I could do, a daring sort of risk-taking for this non-risk-taker. I had a dependable safety net in my purse. My auxiliary mic could polish off the piano noise, and that knowledge made all the difference to me.

Once in my hotel room, and with Ira coming and going for his business meetings, I realized that I should have asked for a telephone alerter. I don't usually put my speech processor on until I get dressed in the morning and Ira has left by then, so I was frequently alone. I knew I missed some phone calls. That was the bad news. The good news was that if the caller left a message, I could retrieve it myself — and I did. I like to use a volume control phone, so that, too, is on my list of things to either bring along or ask for in hotels.

More hotel "non-events" to report. I call attention to these non-events because hearing people don't think anything of them, but if you can't hear, they are embarrassing, frustrating and monumental. Imagine standing in an elevator, somewhere between the first and twentieth floors, and someone comments, "Has it been a good conference for you?" Without hearing, I would have hoped that no one would speak to me in the elevator. And if they did, I might not even have known it. If I did realize someone was speaking to me, I would have either asked them to repeat, saying "Excuse me," or "I'm sorry," or something like that — always apologies — forever apologizing for my lack of hearing. My other option would have been to smile that all-purpose "I have no idea what you said but I hope this lame little smile will make all this (and you) go away quickly." Not exactly conducive to warm human interactions, but a typical fact of life without hearing. Another alternative would have been to explain that I couldn't hear. I never liked that option because the response would inevitably be "Sorry" or a similar expression of condolence, then silence. This would effectively dismiss me as a functioning human being, conveying a "no sense talking to *her*" message.

Someone actually did ask me about the conference while we were riding in the elevator, and I heard them. Instead of using all my wits to get out of a potentially embarrassing situation, I simply responded and even continued the discourse. I told her it was my husband's conference and that I came along to enjoy the sights (and sounds) of Chicago. I then asked her if the conference had been productive for her! What courage this CI gave me! Going even further, I noticed from her name tag that she was also from New Jersey, so I asked her what town she came from. At that point, we had reached the 20th floor, so our conversation ended.

Just comparing the two possible experiences generated by a casual elevator comment — one scenario with hearing, and one without — points up yet again how non-events could be so stressful and potentially mortifying without hearing.

Ira shares my interest in historical sites, so we took a sightseeing side trip to Oak Park, Illinois, a suburb of Chicago, and the first home and studio of architect Frank Lloyd Wright. This was a fascinating place and my first real chance to take a guided tour since getting my CI. In my hearing aid days, when I still had some hearing, I used a personal wireless FM system, giving the microphone and beeper-sized transmitter to the tour guide, and connecting the FM receiver to my hearing aid via a special wire and plug. It had worked well for me when I had no chance of hearing a tour guide otherwise. I can use the same setup with my CI if I want to. The down side is that the guides then expect you to listen to and hear everything they say. Well-intentioned as they might be, sometimes I just don't want to have to deal with that.

This time, with my CI, I wanted to see how I would do on my own. I wore my auxiliary mic and tried to situate myself close to the guide. It was hit and miss, and not just because of me. This guide was pretty old, had a weak voice and missing teeth, so he wasn't the easiest person to understand to begin with. I've learned not to try to hear or even lipread everything from tour guides. It dawned on me a few years ago while touring Chartres Cathedral in France, with its magnificent stained glass windows, that if I spent my time trying to lipread the guide, all my memories would be of the guide's mouth and not the magnificent windows or architecture. So for this tour, once I realized I would get some and miss some, I just relaxed and looked around. There's usually a book in the gift shop describing the exhibit, and we were able to get one on Frank Lloyd Wright's home and studio.

The audio cassette walking tour of the neighborhood, however, was quite another matter! I'm still amazed by the fact that I could even *think* to rent a cassette tour. But I knew from listening to books on tape, especially non-fiction, that I should have no problem understanding it. Cassette tours have always been my favorite, whether for a special museum exhibit or walking the streets of Paris. I love following the directions and listening to the descriptions. It's like a big game with instructions.

The cassette player they offered was an industrial-strength replica of my Sony Walkman. That was a good sign! I brought my own patch cord, plugged in the cassette player on one end and the speech processor on the other, pressed the "PLAY" button — and YES! It was as clear as General Schwarzkopf, Helen Hayes, and Neil Simon narrating their autobiographies. The only difference was those tapes were practice — this was real. I didn't have to "not do something" because of my hearing. If I couldn't have taken the tape tour, I would have missed out on something special. Reading a script would not have been as good because if I was reading, I couldn't be looking at the same time.

We followed the tape — walking to a house, watching and listening, then turning the player off until we headed to the next house. Oak Park has several of Frank Lloyd Wright's earliest home architectural commissions. I was entranced — it was all hearing and I didn't miss a word. What an incredible feeling! Now I know that I can do this in other places as well.

It's ironic that I should do better with these tape systems than with live people, but I know I could even the odds by using a personal FM system with tour guides if I wanted to. The bottom line is to do what I enjoy doing and feel comfortable doing. I just have to remember that I can do this now. Some old "pre-CI, pre-hearing" habits are hard to shake.

DAY 172
MAY 21

My next mapping was supposed to have been in June, six months since getting my speech processor. I scheduled a five-month mapping because I felt that I could be doing better. Even though one of my programs was working for me, I was lured away from it by a stronger program, but I wasn't doing very well in noise with it. At the mapping session, my audiologist checked the settings I was using with the stronger program, and they were no longer correct. I surmise that the very subjective "comfort levels" that are asked for in the mapping process are the key to these settings. I'm never really sure when my "comfortable" is the "comfortable" the manufacturer had in mind.

Three new programs emerged from this mapping, based on slightly changed threshold and comfort levels. Again, the decision had to be made: chuck all the old programs or keep one "tried and true" program. The program I had been favoring was a little too strong and the others were not terrific either, so again I reviewed my new options and made my decision. Chuck 'em all.

If I had written this report a day after that mapping, it would have been filled with frantic ranting and raving. The programs weren't better — they certainly weren't "it." I had been going for better results in noise, and now I wasn't getting better results, period. I was already figuring out how and when to return for a quick visit to my audiologist to get my old program back. And then, a day later, I was okay. Huh? From frantic to fine in twenty-four hours? I'm not one to adjust to change easily (an understatement). I like my old "tried and true," whether a t-shirt or a blanket. I should know by now that this CI hearing process is just not that simple.

I always walk into a mapping session thinking that I'm going to leave with a map that is "better" or "it," but they aren't always instantly better. It reminds me of an allergic reaction that doesn't happen immediately, like eating strawberries but getting hives two days later. It sure would make you wonder what was going on. Similarly, a mapping may not be "good" outside of a quiet one-on-one situation until a day or even a week later.

I should mention that in the testing room, which is quiet one-on-one, I could understand everything without looking using all three programs. From that, I always know that the phone will be okay and so will quiet conversation. Once out of that quiet environment, though, the real world is a much more demanding place.

My auxiliary mic works well for me, but I would still like to do better in noise without it. That explains the push to try new programs even though I still have to remember to give things time. It's not so different from breaking in a new pair of shoes. The new program sounds promising, and I hope to get my brain to work with it and mold it to my liking. I just have to remember that what may ultimately work well for me is not always wonderful on the first day.

DAY 178
MAY 27

My experiences with music continue to puzzle, delight, dismay and evolve. The term "psychophysical" is used to describe the adaptation process the brain goes through in learning to use the CI sound. I'm not an audiologist, but I do know that something strange is going on and I'm still trying to sort it all out. I have been listening to music in a variety of ways although not through my Walkman or Discman yet. (See? I finally learned the official name of the Walkman's disc-playing cousin!) I don't seem to want to listen to music as a main activity, so I usually listen in the car.

What I thought had been my music program, isn't: the one with the random electrode firing order. It must have been a phase I was going through, but whatever sounds it is unscrambling, I don't prefer it to my "main" program anymore.

I had a real surprise the other day — a musical one. I dropped a Glenn Miller tape into my car's tape deck, one I had tried a few months earlier. I remember it sounding so awful, like an ensemble of kazoo-playing mosquitoes. Not pleasant! It didn't take me long to figure out, at the time, that Glenn Miller was going to have to wait. So now, after five months with this CI, I figured I'd give Mr. Miller's music another chance. And it was music this time! "Pennsylvania 6-5000," "In the Mood," I not only could recognize the music, some of it actually sounded pretty good. Not all — the mosquito kazoo band still reigned in a few selections. I'm still trying to figure out which ones and why. I could hear a real big band sound for many of the songs albeit with a froggy quality, as if Louis Armstrong was at the helm. But being able to hear any of the big band sound surprised me because many instruments playing together had been electronic "mush" before. Even in "Pennsylvania 6-5000," where the phone rings — this arrangement used a piano trilling in the high registers — it sounded just like a piano trilling. This was another surprise because pianos still don't usually sound like pianos to me yet.

Why could I now not only recognize but enjoy this tape, which had sounded like garbage just three months before? I could understand if I had "practiced" listening to it, but I hadn't. I had simply stored it away, hoping for "better times" and better sound. And I can't have gotten used to enjoying electronic music mush either — I'm sure of that. And I can't be making this up. I have played this tape over and over because I actually *like* it.

Psychophysics must be at play. This is sort of the opposite of "What you see is what you get." Evidently, what I hear today may not be what I'll be hearing tomorrow. I'm on the lookout now for other surprises.

The piano continues to confound me. Except for that high register trilling I've described, it still sounds very electronic. According to my son, who knows about such things, a piano is one of the most difficult sounds to replicate electronically because of the complex nature of its sound, overtones and other physical properties. It's not that it doesn't sound at all like a piano, it's that it still sounds so electronic — similar to the difference between an electric guitar and an acoustic one.

I keep playing my piano, and listening to a Chopin CD in my car, hoping that my brain will come up with some psychophysical revelation. It may finally be catching on. I was listening to the radio as Ira was driving, so I didn't know what he had tuned into. All of a sudden, my brain said, "That's a piano playing now." I listened some more. "No, brain. That's not a piano — it's some electronic instrument that sounds very remotely like a piano." But my brain insisted, "That is a piano, and whenever you hear that sound, you will think PIANO." I guess all that piano-listening did accomplish something after all. It conditioned me to recognize the sound of a piano, even if it doesn't really sound like one. It's not the worst sound. It just doesn't happen to sound like a piano. But if my brain says this is now what a piano sounds like, I can take the hint.

One "instrument" that does sound "true" is a music box, the sweet tinkle of plucked metallic tones. I bought a lovely little one years ago that plays "It's a Small World," as a souvenir for my children. It looks like a picture frame, with a delightful scene of children dancing, and can be hung on a wall. It has a pull-string, which activates the music box. I bought it to hang near my children's crib and I hadn't seen or heard it in a very long time. I do remember the tinkly tune turning to dull "thumps" as my hearing declined. I don't recall actually putting it away, but it somehow ended up in a box of other useless stuff too good to discard.

I'm not sure why I found this music box at this particular time, (a little metaphysics at play here?) but when I saw it, I knew I had to try listening to it again. As I pulled the string, not knowing what I would hear — kazoo-playing mosquitoes, an electronic simulation, or the real thing — a rush of memories flooded back. I had always liked that music box, and particularly that song. CI's and Swiss music box movements must be made for each other because the bell-like tinkle was almost exactly as I remembered it. Now, I hope my family will bear with me as I listen to "It's a Small World" for the hundredth time.

DAY 179
MAY 28

I've been listening to my Glenn Miller tape again and again. Some of it is divine — some of it is not. I'm also experiencing something especially bizarre, something I didn't expect. There is a string bass accompaniment throughout most of the numbers, a constant thump, thump, thump, thump, thump, thump, thump. But I'm not hearing it with my CI speech processor. I'm hearing it with my *unimplanted* ear while listening to it in my car stereo. I didn't think my right ear, which doesn't even have a hearing aid in it, could hear anything anymore. Just when you think you have life figured out, it gives you a little surprise like that. But that string bass accompaniment is all that it is hearing, none of the rest of the music. I must have more low frequency hearing, lower than they check on hearing tests, than I thought.

I'm not hearing the string bass with my CI, so it's almost like stereo — deep bass in the unimplanted ear, everything else in the CI ear. This is a fascinating and efficient use of all my hearing in a most pleasant way! I keep talking about how music with a CI doesn't sound like normal hearing, but hearing the "real" string bass sound anchors me somehow. That must explain why I enjoy listening to this tape over and over again. It's probably one of the only styles of music that I could do this with, and I have a sneaking suspicion my brain knows it too. It keeps asking for more.

It sometimes makes a difference to listen for a while before giving up on something harsh-sounding. A case in point is in temple. I'm told the Cantor has a lovely voice, but it definitely sounds more melodic after I listen for a while. I'm not sure what the explanation is. I think that my brain is molding what I am hearing into its own mental memory of what it should sound like. So I'm learning to be patient, not rejecting anything right away.

I tried this theory on my Bach organ music CD and, unfortunately, I'm convinced that I'm still not ready for that type of music. Goodness knows what sort of sound waves organs make, but my speech processor is simply not ready to interpret it for me. I'll just have to wait.

The *Nutcracker Suite* is another story. I played through several sections of the suite, giving it all a chance, and concluded that some of it was not only recognizable, but even pleasant. The "Overture" wasn't bad and the "March" was better. The celeste, an instrument featured in one of the sections, almost sounds the way it should — a lovely bell-like quality. The "Waltz of the Flowers" won this contest, though, possibly because of the emphasis on the brass instruments, which came in well. And I'm finding myself playing the harp solo over and over again. I really enjoy listening to it — I guess, because it sounds like a harp!

Another aspect of music appreciation that I didn't expect was its effect on my dancing. As my hearing bowed out, I lost the desire to dance. I thought it might have had something to do with the aging process, but I don't think so anymore. I was at two bar mitzvahs this month and I danced up a storm. Hearing the music is definitely more conducive to dancing than just hearing the thuds of the rhythm, which was all I could hear before my CI. This must relate to coordinating dance movements with the sound of the music. Just hearing or feeling the rhythm doesn't have the same effect. I really thought it was my thick head and leaden feet that were keeping me from Electric Sliding and macarena-ing. NO! It was the lack of melody reaching my brain. So now I'm relieved to find out that my brain, when it is inspired by some melody, is happy to tell my feet what to do.

And speaking of bar mitzvahs, I could actually hear part of the services even though neither temple had an infrared system. I even laughed at one of the rabbi's jokes as he spoke to my nephew, Mark, praising the fine rendition of his Haftorah "without breaking a sweat." A lot of people laughed out loud. But when I laughed out loud, it drew comments from my husband and my son. They hadn't heard me laugh like that — with everybody else — in a very long time, possibly ever. People who are hard of hearing don't usually laugh with everyone else. I would have to ask what was so funny and then have it explained to me later. And "later," a joke is never funny enough to laugh at. This is yet another facet of hearing loss that nobody talks about, the isolation of not being able to laugh along with others. It had never seemed particularly important to me before although I did know the hurt feelings of being shut out like that. But it was important enough for both my husband and son to comment about, that I could understand a joke and laugh. With that bittersweet revelation, yet another little piece of me emerges.

DAY 187
JUNE 5

After six months, I'm still experiencing that "better" syndrome that "they" said would keep happening. I was at a meeting at the League for the Hard of Hearing, with about 20 people around a conference table, and I gave a short presentation. I heard a question from the other end of the table, while looking at the person, and I thought that was pretty good. But then, out of somewhere, I heard another question — a follow-up to the previous one — and, without a moment's hesitation, I answered that one too. But I immediately realized that I didn't know who had asked me the question. That doesn't happen to me, or at least it never happened to me before. And, in the next instant, someone who was out of my view, hidden behind another person's head, shot his hand up, poked his face out, and said that he had asked the question!

This was *really* a new one on me; not only that I could hear the question without looking, but that my brain heard the question, understood the question, and responded to the question, without "trying." And this questioner was almost at the other end of the table. I felt as if I had been struck by lightning, clear out of the blue. This is definitely an example of doing "better!"

I seem to be turning to music more and more — not on an experimental basis, but to actually enjoy it. The first six months must be characterized as "the beginning" with all the trials and errors and figuring out what is going on here. Now, I'm starting to enjoy more and "figure" less.

I went to a choral concert, complete with chamber orchestra. My friend, Susan, was singing, and asked me if I'd like to attend. I had been practicing listening to orchestral and choral music, so I felt ready to go to a concert for enjoyment, and not just for experimentation. From my tape and CD-listening experiences, I had a pretty good idea of what instruments sound most "true" and which don't. I was curious about hearing these instruments "live," and with Susan singing in the chorus, that was just the incentive I needed.

Some philosophy enters this picture: that the glass is half-full and not half-empty. It would be very easy to get into a "half-empty" mindset while listening to music with my CI. There's plenty that doesn't sound the way it used to. But I have progressed, through time and practice, to the stage where music is discernible as music. It didn't all start out that way. Some of it was electronic mush, a quality which had me reaching for the "off" switch. I'm not finding that to be the case anymore.

True to my expectations, the live instruments at the concert came through as they did on my recordings. The "half-full" roster of instruments that sound pretty much as they should are basically the wind instruments: oboe, flute, bassoon, clarinet, and brass. The bassoon, English horn and trombone are the winners right now. Being at a live concert, I had a better chance to identify the strings individually, and as I expected, violins are in the "half-empty" category. They still sound screechy and shrill. Cellos aren't bad, though — a lot better than the violins. And violas and the lowest string of the violin resemble string sound. By going in person to a concert, I could see who was playing and identify the sounds more easily than just by listening to the recordings.

Among the voices, the basses and tenors were best, with altos okay, and sopranos rather shrill. Why high-pitched sounds, like violins and sopranos, are unpleasant, but flutes, which are also high-pitched, are fine is still a mystery. The biggest hurdle in listening to a concert with voices and orchestra playing together was that it could easily have turned into "mush." But it didn't and I had a feeling that it wouldn't.

It is a slow progression, but I suspected reaching a new level because I'm gravitating to music in my car. I could easily reach for the news or weather, or an audio book, but I keep coming back to music. I wouldn't be doing that if the sound was torturous.

I headed back to the record store for CD's and tapes that I thought I would hear best. This reminds me of selecting shoes, clothing, or even golf clubs according to what "fits" best — so why not music too? That's where the "half-full" philosophy kicks in. If I can be happy with at least some of the music, and not dwell on the negatives, that's good. Very good. After all, how did Caruso sound on those early Victrolas? And people thought *that* was fabulous! Same idea. It's a whole lot better than not hearing any music at all.

DAY 208
JUNE 26

This week was the week of the dentists — starting on Monday with my regular dentist, graduating to a periodontist, and then finally to an endodontist. I have never had problems with my teeth, so this was all new to me. Approaching any doctor's office always filled me with dread and a heightened sense of alert, not only because of a medical problem, but because trying to hear in those environments was always fraught with tension, stress, and fear of the unknown. Incredibly, this whole dental episode, which should have been so unpleasant, ended up being another "CI moment."

It's hard to fathom how much difference being able to hear can make in almost every situation, and dentists' offices are another case in point. Beginning with the initial "complaint" phone call, I knew immediately this was going to be different. I placed the call, and talking to the receptionist to make an appointment was a breeze! She was wondering how I had made a regular voice call because she had always fielded my Relay calls in the past. I let her know what was new: with my CI, I can use a regular voice phone.

Sitting in a dentist's chair was always difficult for me. People would approach from behind — talking, asking questions. The usual dentist's set-up was never conducive to easy communication for someone who needed to lipread to understand. The dentist would probe, and then turn aside to make notes. This time, there was no problem. I didn't have to remind them to face me. Even when I didn't have full view, it was trouble-free communication.

Granted, it was my best kind of environment — quiet, with people at close range. But that was the case before too, and it was always so stressful.

Next stop was the periodontist. Evidently, even with teeth, everyone's a specialist. I should mention that with each new medical practitioner, I pulled out my CI Patient Information card to show what precautions needed to be taken in medical treatment with an implant. They would usually make a copy of this and put it in my file. As I sat in the waiting room, I was not nervous at all about hearing my name being called. I didn't have to scan the desk area constantly. I just sat back and read my *People* magazine. If you see enough doctors, there's no need ever to get a subscription to *People* magazine. I always look forward to this treat, something trivial and light while waiting to have my mouth probed.

At this dentist's office, I chatted for a while with the dental assistant. No problems there as she x-rayed, moved around the chair and did all sorts of things behind my back. I knew what was going on. No stress — although I was a little curious (make that a *lot* curious) to see if I could function without asking for repeats or to see their faces. Communication wasn't all out of my sight — it was just normal movement — and I was able to do it. Yes, I asked for some repeats, but not many.

Not to go into the details of my dental problems, it turned out that I had to be referred to yet another dentist, an endodontist. As often happens in medical offices, I was standing at the reception area with the periodontist as he was speaking on the phone to the endodontist, asking him if he could see me right away. I followed his end of the conversation and I noted that he was now talking to the receptionist, setting up an appointment for me. He then handed me the phone, telling me to arrange a convenient time to come in.

I looked at the phone. It looked back at me, and my life flashed before my eyes. I had been in this situation so many times before. I could never use a phone handed to me like that. Initially, when my hearing was not too bad, I still needed a volume control receiver, which these office phones never had. And later, when I couldn't use a voice phone anymore, it became impossible to use a phone handed to me in a medical office like that. So we're talking about 25 years of having to ask for assistance with the phone in this situation.

I stared at the phone. I knew that it was a regular phone, without a volume control. I also knew that the office reception area was not absolutely quiet. There was a general hum of people talking and going about their work. Background noise has been a problem for me on the phone, so I had my doubts about how well I would hear. It seemed like forever before I took that receiver and held it up to my CI mic. I didn't even think about what it looked like to the others standing there since, of course, I didn't put it on my ear. Everyone was to my right, and my head mic is on my left side, so I guess it looked pretty normal from where they were standing.

I said hello, wondering what would happen. And then the receptionist on the other end of the line came in loud and clear — bless her soul! I stood there, arranging to come in at 12. Yes, I could make it a little earlier — 11:30 was okay. Yes, I knew how to get to their office. See you later. And I hung up.

I have been writing these chronicles for over six months now, and I know how other people have cried when they see me hearing again or when they talk to me on the phone. My own reaction has always been joy — pure joy — not tears. Let me tell you, this time I had tears in my eyes. This was overwhelming. This was not a practice phone call. This wasn't under optimum conditions. This was real life. The dentist handed me the phone, treating me like a hearing person, and I stood there talking on the phone like a hearing person.

It was a little bizarre, welling up with tears of joy after making arrangements for yet another dental appointment, something not usually rejoiced over. Interestingly, the dental assistant came over to me. She had been concerned when she saw the dentist hand the phone over to me. She knew about my CI (as did the dentist) and she was ready to assist if need be. I don't know if this was doctor/nurse or male/female behavior at play. But it was obvious that it never crossed the dentist's mind that I might not be able to hear on the phone. Then again, I guess I'd rather have him worrying about my gums than my telephone abilities. I already have a specialist for that!

Next stop was the endodontist and the whole receptionist scene was repeated. I ended up in yet another dentist's chair, again explaining my CI and showing my CI information card with its precautions. And again, the dentist and assistants were coming and going, turning away, writing — and I was following along, entranced and amazed. I wasn't struggling to understand and I didn't have to keep reminding people to look at me or slow down. I think I asked for some repeats, but if I can't really remember, then it couldn't have been many.

The diagnosis was "root canal," and the endodontist put on his little surgical mask, the kind that makes any lipreader's heart sink. I waited, and listened, and I could not believe it, but I heard him right through that mask. Yes, I would have preferred to see his mouth, but I heard the instructions and I heard him behind my back, too. Rinse, open wider, etc. (I'll spare you the details of root canal instructions.)

It was a weird situation. I was in a dentist's chair having root canal, and I was absolutely thrilled to hear what was going on. I think the dentist was a little surprised at how happy I was. This certainly couldn't have been the norm. And another emotion emerged — something that was gradually surfacing as this whole tooth drama was unfolding — that I could concentrate on the medical problem and not have to use all my wits and energy to understand what was going on. A huge hurdle had been removed. We could just talk about teeth, not hearing.

Always, always, always, whenever I had anything to do with health care — whether in doctor's offices or in hospitals — it was always about hearing, no matter why I was there. This was so different; I didn't have to preface every motion with warnings about how best to communicate with me. And even that surgical mask experience brought back memories. A few years ago, I had been in an operating suite, unable to understand a word because of those masks. I faced the dilemma of having them pull the masks down so I could see their mouths and understand their instructions, risking contamination — or letting them leave their masks in place, not understanding a word and hoping for the best. Those experiences leave emotional scars and they have stayed with me.

I can't say that root canal was the most pleasant of experiences and I'm not in a big rush to have any more, but compared to doing any medical procedure without hearing, it was a breeze.

DAY 224
JULY 12

I've always loved visiting historic houses or opulent mansions from the past, so Ira and I found ourselves at Skylands Manor and Botanical Gardens in northern New Jersey, a place we'd never been to before. The grounds of this mansion were laid out as formal and informal gardens, with walking paths, fountains, statues — the works! Strolling through gardens has always been an enjoyable activity for me because no hearing was necessary. I could see, smell and touch the flowers.

As we walked along the formal gardens near the main house, I noticed that the fountains were not silent. The water bubbled, trickled, spouted, splashed — all verbs that conjured up visual images, but now took on additional meanings of *sound*. This caught me off guard. Fountains had always been lovely to look at but now were delightful to hear. I was acting like a curious little child again. Ira wanted to keep walking. I wanted to stay and listen. The water lapped over a ledge, gurgling as it dropped into a lily-pad pool below. I hadn't heard that sound in a very long time.

We left the formal garden area and went to the Bog Garden, a quiet pond strewn with water lilies, the kind that had inspired Monet to greatness. Everything was very still and beautiful — a natural setting — different from the formal gardens we had just left. And then Ira said, "Listen." Ira has never said "listen" to me before, not on these nature walks. He's always pointed, not even bothering to say "look at this" because I wouldn't have heard that either. We had developed a "point and look" system of communication out of habit and necessity. But now, I was told to "listen" — and I could.

I heard croaks — very soft croaks. There were frogs in that Bog Garden. We looked closer, and sure enough, there they were! I heard a foghorn sort of noise and Ira told me that was a bullfrog, sitting up on a lily-pad. We stood still and listened to this symphony of frogs, all croaking to each other. What a delightful chorus! This was so new to me — sharing the sounds of nature, not just the sights or smells. I felt as if Mother Nature had beckoned me here, just to witness this wonder of sound.

Back home, I've noticed that I'm understanding the television better, even my big-screen tv at a distance. We were watching "60 Minutes," and I hadn't bothered to put on the captioning yet when I noticed that I was understanding what they were saying. Hmmm... and the sound from that distance wasn't as hoarse as it had been. Something had changed, and it wasn't my speech processor because I haven't had a mapping in over a month. I think it was a "brain thing" again. "60 Minutes" is usually easier to follow than most programming because they do full-face interviews, so there is ample opportunity to lipread as well. But I was never very good at lipreading people on tv. This was definitely an improvement in hearing skills.

So, what did I do next? I tuned into the "Three Tenors" concert broadcast from the Eiffel Tower in Paris, without captions. I had enjoyed listening to a Pavarotti tape recently, so this particular broadcast caught my interest. This was actually a two-part experiment. Could I hear the tenors as music, and could I understand the narration without captions (and without a face to lipread)? The answers: pretty much and pretty much. (No, nothing is perfect these days — everything with a grain of salt.) This was the first time I had listened to music on my television and it wasn't bad. It was about the same as my other music experiences: the first impression of the music was electronic and then, as I gave my brain a chance to get used to the sound, it became more melodic and natural. I understood more of the narration, without lipreading or captions, than I ever expected. I didn't want to turn it off! No doubt about it — this was definitely "better."

And as an encore to this report: Ira and I went out for an evening stroll with our friends, Joan and Marty, on a dark, unlit path. As I walked along with Joan, we chatted, both of us looking straight ahead. Without my saying a word about my hearing, Joan said to me, "I can't believe we're walking along talking in the dark!" It's one thing for me to notice changes in my life because of my new hearing, but I forget sometimes how much my lack of hearing had an impact on others and how they had to accommodate themselves just to communicate with me. It wasn't only easier for me to hear my friend now, it was easier for her to be with me too. Even in the dark of night, the clouds had parted and the sunshine was streaming in.

DAY 229
JULY 17

I went to my temple's Annual Sisterhood Pool Party this week, an event I hadn't gone to in several years. As my hearing declined, it had become too difficult to attend an event that was supposed to be fun, but was just torture for me. I vividly remember the last time, sitting at a picnic table, unable to follow the lively conversations around me. As I became bored and started daydreaming (I had to do something with my brain!), I noticed that people at my table had stopped talking and were staring at me. I had that uneasy "I have no idea what is going on now" feeling, and saw some nervous giggles. I figured that someone must have been talking to me. This particular table of people did not know about my hearing loss, so they didn't realize that I hadn't heard them. I set them straight, and they were all good-natured about it and happy to assist me, but it was an embarrassing, uncomfortable ordeal. Right then and there I decided that I didn't need this kind of "fun."

So, it's been a while since I've gone to a pool party. I was really looking forward to this one because even if I didn't know all the women, I could at least talk to them, now that I could hear. I skipped the water aerobics because I didn't want to be deaf again at one of these affairs. I chatted instead with another landlubber, and munched and sipped. I wanted to see if I could understand in the noise of this party without my auxiliary mic. Talking one-on-one, with the sound of the water aerobics music and chatter in the background, I was fine with my "noise program." Once all the women were sitting around the tables and babbling non-stop, I couldn't hear the individual voices any more. This is my most difficult hearing environment — a lot of voices in close range of my head mic. They all blur together.

Once I put the auxiliary mic on, I was fine and could hear pretty well at the luncheon table. I'm figuring out that by using the auxiliary mic, it positions a microphone where the people I want to hear are — not behind my ear, but in front of me. It was evident that there was not going to be any repeat of that embarrassing silence I had experienced at the last pool party. I felt as if I was getting back into the saddle after being thrown from my horse, but with new and improved protective gear — hearing!

The ladies were selling raffle tickets for the door prizes and when it came to deciding how many tickets to buy — 3 for $5 or 8 for $10 — I looked in my wallet, saw that I didn't have any five dollar bills and would need change if I only bought three tickets. I figured that I hadn't been to one of these parties in several years, and it was all for a good cause, so I bought $10's worth, making up for lost time.

Buying raffle tickets had an added perspective for me. I knew that I would be able to hear them announce the winning numbers this time. I wouldn't have to ask someone to check my numbers to see if I had won. There were only about twenty women there and most were buying three tickets each. Since I was buying more tickets than anyone else, I figured I had a pretty good chance of winning at least one of the three door prizes, which were sitting on the table, all wrapped up.

The first number was picked. I heard it, looked down at my numbers — and I won! I had my choice of the three gifts, and I picked the smallest package. Since I was the winner, I had the privilege of picking the next ticket. I closed my eyes, rummaged through the bowl, and picked the next winner. I looked down, called out the number and realized that I had won AGAIN! "Am I allowed to win twice?" I asked. "Sure, why not," was the reply. I guess my decision to buy more tickets than anyone else *had* improved my chances of winning. I picked the smaller of the two remaining prizes and then waited for the next number to be called. I heard the last winning number, but it wasn't one of mine. I was happy to see someone else know the thrill of hearing a winning number.

Everyone wanted to see what I had won, so I opened the gifts right then and there. The first one, the smallest, was a glass bud vase — a nice prize. The next gift was a little bigger, and felt like two items. Pulling off the outer wrap, then the tissue paper, it was, indeed, two items — a box of note-cards and a picture frame. The notecards had an artistic drawing of a cochlea-shaped shell on the front, with the words "LISTEN CLOSELY" printed around it. The picture frame was decorated with a spiral shell design. I looked at the notecards not knowing what to think. Even as I type this, it feels as if I am writing a novel — something surrealistic — but this is exactly what happened. I am not making this up.

This "event" deserved an explanation, so I made an "acceptance" speech, showing and telling about my cochlear implant and my new-found hearing. I also pointed out that I hadn't picked those notecards, with their all-too-perfect design and inscription, until I had won the second time. I asked the person who bought the door prizes why she had picked these items, hoping to find some explanation for this "coincidence." She said, no, she did-n't have any premonitions about buying those particular items. She had always liked shells.

And that is the story of the Sisterhood Pool Party. Was it a "religious experience" or just a coincidence? I write this with no commentary. I leave it for you to ponder.

DAY 256
AUGUST 13

Every summer, my friends from the Costume Restoration Group of the Hermitage historic house in HoHoKus, New Jersey, visit the summer home of Jeanette, one of our "Sewing Ladies." I have been joining this group up to the lake house for the past five years and, as you can imagine, it had become more and more difficult to have "fun" at this annual outing. Last year was very difficult, as I watched the lively discussions and laughter around me, unable to follow much of it.

This year was totally different. "The Ladies" already knew that I could hear, but Jeanette's husband, Bert, hadn't seen me since last summer. Bert is an 88-year-old retired minister with a charming personality. As soon as we pulled up in their driveway and walked up the path to their house, he greeted me with, "There's my miracle girl!" and a warm hug.

As the afternoon progressed, Bert couldn't get over how different I was. He said that last year, I just sat there politely "like a bump on a log," but now I was so actively part of the conversation, laughing and happy. We talked about miracles, and he said this was an absolute miracle. It was nice getting a professional's opinion!

Not only was the afternoon pleasant, getting there and coming home were also wonderful. I was driving and could understand my friend sitting next to me even though she was on my "worse" side. We chatted back and forth non-stop the entire way, over an hour each way — quite a difference from driving in silence I had become accustomed to!

My Supermarket Sagas continue as well. I've reported before how the little things can sometimes make such a big difference. This time I was reaching for some dental floss on an upper shelf, and in the process, set off an avalanche of Tylenol. I heard the woman standing next to me comment, "This place must be booby-trapped!" I turned around, laughing, and told her I thought so too. And in the back of my mind, I noted that here I was laughing and enjoying a spontaneous comment because I could hear, knowing full well that this would have been another embarrassing moment if I couldn't. I might not have turned around; she would have wondered why I didn't respond; I might have smiled lamely and nervously because of the way she would have been looking at me. That scenario was all too familiar to me. It was a welcome relief to be able to laugh instead.

Come to think of it, I seem to be laughing a *lot* more. And smiling too. Again in the supermarket, I heard my name called from behind, and there was an old friend from high school, who happens to live in my town. I walked right over, and through the beep-beeps of the supermarket checkout lines, we caught up on some family doings. This wouldn't have happened at all before. I would never have heard her calling me, and I sure wouldn't have wanted to chat in the supermarket because I would never have understood her. Avoiding personal contact — that's what I had always done pre-CI. Not anymore, at least not because of my hearing.

And it happened again, just the other day. I met someone in the supermarket who said hello to me, but I didn't recognize him. It turned out to be my friend Susan's husband whom I had only met briefly at one of his wife's choral concerts. We chatted briefly and then went on our way. This *never* would have happened pre-CI. It would have been another embarrassing "get me out of here" moment!

I'm also revisiting experiences that I've already had with my CI. Remember the last time I was at Yankee Stadium, on Opening Day, and I was disappointed not to be able to hear Robert Merrill singing — it all sounded like echo-y mush? Well, back into the Stadium for Old Timers' Day, three months later, I was all prepared to be disappointed again as Robert Merrill stepped up to the microphone. Lo and behold, I heard him singing "America the Beautiful" even in that cavernous stadium with the echo-y sound! The magic of CI progress continues!

And last on my list: I was in Chicago again for a few days. Chicago is known for its architecture, and the Chicago Architecture Foundation gives wonderful walking tours. I really wanted to go on a tour, so I signed up for one — and, yes, I heard the guide as we walked along the noisy streets of Chicago. I put my "noise" program on, although I could have used my auxiliary mic too. I was lipreading about 30% and hearing the rest. But the point of the matter is that I wouldn't have contemplated taking a walking tour before. Not a chance! This turned out to be a lot of fun, and I even talked to some of the other people on my tour — like a real person.

DAY 269
AUGUST 26

If you can stand yet another episode of my Supermarket Sagas, I finally got a chance to test out the "bakery numbers" at the deli counter. Before my CI, that was one place that I had learned from bitter experience to avoid. In order to respond promptly to the numbers they were calling, I had to watch the people behind the counter — often two or three people moving back and forth — because they would frequently call out the numbers before advancing the electronic sign. I had suffered the embarrassment of responding to the posted number, only to learn that they had already called my number and several after mine before advancing the numbers. So, once again, I had become an animal on the prowl, watching every move. The "reward" for responding correctly was to try and lipread the person behind the counter. It just wasn't worth it for half a pound of Swiss cheese!

With my CI, I've gone back to using deli counters again, but for some reason, I hadn't encountered the "bakery numbers" until just the other day. No sweat — I was a seasoned enough CI-user to know that this should not present a problem. I took number 92, and they were already up to 89, so it was not going to be a long wait. I stood there, not really focusing on anything in particular, when I heard the woman behind the counter call 90, 91, 92. And with 92, I held up my hand and gave her my order. Never in my life was ordering a pound of honey-roasted turkey breast so easy! As I pushed my shopping cart away, ready to continue my shopping, my brain started giving me an argument — "That's it? We don't have to stalk this place, use all our wits to jump in at the right time? When do we get to use all our wits,

Arlene?!" I really felt this sense of expectation — I was so conditioned to ready myself for the "battle." But if you can hear the numbers, and hear the person behind the counter, it's a rather simple task, instead of being a minefield of stress.

I spent an evening out with my daughter, Emily, and two of her friends. I had never been able to chat with any of her friends before my CI. There was never any point asking them questions because I knew I wouldn't understand the answers. Whenever conversations were directed my way, Emily would have to "interpret" for me. I could understand her, but not her friends. So as far as they were concerned, they never knew me. I wasn't much more than wallpaper to them.

The evening I spent with Emily and her friends was an experience I had never known. I asked them questions — they answered me. I found out what their plans were, what they did for the summer, when they were going back to school. We went to a show, so we discussed the production — the nuances of the sets, the actors, everything. As we drove in the car, I could understand Emily sitting next to me, and some of what the other two girls were saying behind me. I couldn't follow their fast-paced three-way conversation, but I could catch bits and pieces — sometimes enough to ask a question to remain involved.

I had a real surprise, though, when we were stopped at a red light on our way home. As the light changed to green and I got ready to put my foot on the accelerator, I heard a little voice from behind say, "Green light!" I almost laughed out loud. My first backseat driver! I never had one before. I had started to lose my hearing at about the same time that I had gotten my driver's license, almost 30 years ago. I have never heard any comments from the backseat and only a few from the passenger side, but even those petered out eventually. Backseat drivers — another CI milestone!

DAY 276
SEPTEMBER 2

I have just finished putting the invitations in the mail for the League for the Hard of Hearing's annual Comedy Night. This is one of the League's big fundraisers, but it is also the only chance to enjoy a night of stand-up comedy at a real New York Comedy Club, Caroline's, with an infrared system, realtime captioning and sign language interpreters. This is our eleventh year going, and we've been on the Comedy Night Planning Committee for almost as many years. As I sent off those envelopes, I couldn't help but remember the emotions attached to Comedy Nights past, and how this one, with my new-found CI hearing would be different.

The degenerative nature of my hearing loss always hit home with these annual events. Without fail, I always heard less than the year before, and Comedy Nights were another benchmark in my hearing decline. I remember when I was able to use the infrared system alone quite successfully. But with each successive year I had less hearing, so I had to sit closer to the front to read the comedians' lips. Then I needed the volume boosted to the maximum. Finally, they started realtime captioning the event, which was a relief because, by then, I wouldn't have been able to understand anything without it.

With each passing year, the entourage of friends and colleagues joining us for this night of fun has kept growing — wonderfully so! Two years ago, about a week before the event, my hearing took another dive, and my hearing aid's little auxiliary microphone — my lifeline — was no longer working for me. Panic set in because we had about 75 people coming to join us for what was supposed to be an evening of fun. The League came to the rescue (once again) and quickly fixed me up with a stronger auxiliary microphone, and that seemed to work. At least I could hear *something*, and I was able to get through the evening.

Last year, with over 90 people to meet and greet, even the most powerful auxiliary microphone wasn't helping. At that point, I was looking forward to my CI surgery, but I still had to function with the events in my life until then. To socialize with that many people with virtually no hearing and no practice at that level was a monumental challenge, especially to keep smiling.

The strategy for that evening was the "pounce" technique. (Those who have done this know what I'm talking about. Those who are struggling may find this helpful. Those who have been pounced, at least now you will know what hit you.) This strategy involved greeting people and starting the conversation *before* they had a chance to talk. Controlling the conversation, the topic, the pleasantries — that was the only way to get through socializing with so many people with virtually no hearing. I did that for an hour, and then laughed at the stand-up comedians by following the captioning and lipreading. I always figured that if I laughed at even one joke, it was more laughter than I would have had sitting home. And this time I laughed more than once, so it was all worthwhile, and the League raised a lot of needed funds.

This year, I'm hoping that even more people will turn out. And I'm not in a panic now worrying about my hearing getting worse, or having to get more powerful microphones that may or may not work for me. This time, I have my CI, and even though I know I'll be using the auxiliary mic to hear better in the noisy "meet and greet" environment, I know that (barring any technical snafus!), it will deliver the sound. As for the comedians: I'm going to be using the infrared system with the captions as backup, and if they talk right into the microphone as they usually do, I should be in good shape. My hunch is that the smiles will come a lot easier and I may even let someone else "pounce" first.

DAY 296
SEPTEMBER 22

I've had my CI for almost ten months now, so I'm still experiencing events that happen only once a year. These past two days were Rosh Hashannah, and although I had already been to my synagogue several times with my CI, the liturgy of this holiday and the rituals, customs and memories made for another unique experience. I've said before that each annual event always served as a benchmark for my deteriorating hearing — each year being worse than the year before — and each year brought its next round of coping strategies and electronic equipment to keep me functioning.

Last year at this time, I had almost completed the evaluation for my CI, and my hearing was all but gone. I had always used the infrared system in my synagogue, even when it barely did any good, but last year I didn't even bother. The sound it brought in was harsh and useless. I resolved to just sit there, following what I could and steeping myself in private thought. Ira, whom I could lipread without sound, would oral interpret the Rabbi's sermon for me. He didn't always do it verbatim, and although I asked him to give me "just the facts," he would editorialize. I couldn't fault him for that. It was a strenuous exercise to listen, then mouth the words of the entire sermon. I was grateful to him, but I found it hard to have to rely on others to understand what was going on.

I have a wonderful friend, Judy, in my congregation who had offered to sign interpret or oral interpret for me. I declined both offers, not that I wouldn't have wanted to take her up on them. I don't know sign language (except for the Girl Scout Promise, from my tenure as Troop Leader

— not terribly useful in practical life.) My lipreading skills were good enough to lipread my husband without sound, but not many other people.

Chatting with the other members of the congregation was difficult, if not impossible. The choir, which performs at only a few services, appeared to be singing nicely, fervently for all I knew — but to me it was just noise. I was shut out of just about everything everyone else was hearing or doing. The one thing I did have last year, as bad as my hearing had gotten, was HOPE.

This year, of course, was different — very different. I had expectations because after so many months with my CI, I knew pretty much what I could do and what I couldn't. I started by trying to listen to the service without the infrared, and I could actually hear much more than I expected. Temple Beth Or's sanctuary is quite large, with high ceilings, so the sound had a bit of an echo, and I couldn't understand without looking. Once I plugged my speech processor into the infrared receiver, voices were crisp and clear. I sat and listened — to the Rabbi, to the Cantor, to the choir. Each had a microphone nearby, so the sound was not distorted. Recalling my "Gold, Silver, and Bronze" hearing categories, I would say that what had been Silver hearing before in this situation — that is, the ability to understand speech without looking, but the meaning still being processed separately — had moved up to Gold in this very controlled environment. I felt that as well as I had done before, I was doing even better now. Hear/Understand — very little "processing" was necessary, and that was real progress.

It still amazed me, though, as I sat there, listening to the familiar sounds around me, just what it was taking to allow me to hear! I am deaf! Without any electronics, I hear *nothing*! Plugged into the infrared system, I could hear every rustle of paper, every "s" and "t" the Rabbi uttered, every tone of the Cantor's chant. I kept imagining the sound, being beamed via infrared light, entering my speech processor and being converted to a signal that would control the firing of those electrodes in my cochlea. How this could ever be real continues to remain a mystery, and can still only be called a miracle.

As *Avenu Malkeinu*, the traditional Rosh Hashannah prayer and chant, was intoned by the Cantor and the chorus, tears welled up in my eyes. My friends in the choir knew that I had loved their singing but had been unable to hear them last year. I heard them. Again, it happened that the music sounded better the longer I listened. After about 45 minutes, my brain became used to the melodious harmonies of the choir and the Cantor. Although they still had an electronic tinge, the chants were definitely familiar and, in their own way, beautiful — perhaps even more beautiful than those hearing it through normal ears.

I attended two services for Rosh Hashannah, Sunday evening and Monday morning. With both of my children home for the holidays, we got off to a late start Monday morning and arrived at temple a few minutes after the services had started. We had *never* been late before — never. As we entered the lobby area, we heard the service being broadcast over a loudspeaker — "I, the Lord, am your God, who led you out of Egypt to be your God; I, the Lord, am your God." Quite a way to be greeted! I suspect I am not alone in my thoughts about Divine intervention when it comes to CI's. There is no way to escape these thoughts when contemplating the miracle I have been experiencing. Hearing this part of the service broadcast over the loudspeaker, so unexpectedly, made me pause. I had wandered in the desert of hearing loss for thirty years.

My hearing on the second day was about the same as the first. I can't say whether it took me less time to adjust to the music, but I was definitely getting used to being there — all of me. One thing that had remained the same as in the past was that I didn't sing along or recite the prayers aloud with everyone else. Being plugged into the infrared system, I couldn't hear my own voice because the system only brings in the sound picked up by the microphones. I had always been afraid of speaking too loud, or singing off-key, so even yesterday I didn't participate — *until* — it dawned on me that no matter what I sounded like, it didn't really matter. Not only that, I realized that I *should* recite the prayers with everyone else, even if I couldn't tell how loudly I was speaking. And I *should* sing along too. So by the end of the second service, I was participating again — hearing the Rabbi, the Cantor, the choir — but not myself. Singing along was a little strange. I found myself adjusting my voice to keep in tune, whatever that means. I have no idea if I was singing in tune, but my brain was definitely trying to control my vocal chords. How this was happening — again, I don't know. No one looked at me funny, so I guess I was doing all right. I had this content little feeling, though, that *whatever* I did, I had this special "right" to do it. I had been blessed with this CI miracle, and one doesn't argue with miracles, especially in synagogues.

One difference I hadn't expected was during the blowing of the shofar, the ram's horn. Even last year, I could hear that sound, but it was harsh to my ears. I remember having to turn down the volume on my hearing aid to listen to it. This year, it wasn't the same at all. The sound was lovely, controlled, but not overly loud. I didn't cringe. I enjoyed it. I could simply take it all in, calmly and serenely, something I hadn't been able to do in many years.

After the services, I had a chance to chat with friends. When they were talking about the Rabbi's sermon, some people said they had trouble catching one of the punch lines of a story he had told. Evidently, they were having difficulty with the phrase "think of the odds." I had no trouble understanding the Rabbi at all, and I verified what they thought he had said. Perhaps bionic hearing, especially plugged into an infrared system, does put one at an advantage over hearing mortals. I'm starting to sound a little too smug, because the truth of the matter is that this entire temple experience was humbling. I had always prayed for the strength to be able to cope with my hearing loss, but to have my prayers answered like this is simply beyond my comprehension.

DAY 309
OCTOBER 5

My most recent report about Rosh Hashannah generated many comments, more than anything else I've written. I don't feel it's fair to keep these to myself. Actually, I've been receiving comments all along about my experiences, and I'd like to share a few of those with you, too. Once you read them, I think you'll understand why I've kept writing.

Responding to my Rosh Hashannah report, two people struggling with hearing loss had this to say:

> "*I relate to everything you felt a year ago because that's exactly the state I'm in now with my progressive hearing loss. . . . With God's good blessing, I'll be in your shoes this time next year.*"
>
> Janet T.

> "*I am greatly encouraged by your experience in temple. I have not attended services myself in a couple of years because of an inability to hear well enough. Your experience has given me a sense of hope.*"
>
> Bernard K.

Those who already had CI's had a different perspective on my Rosh Hashannah report:

> "Your eloquent story echoes my thoughts and feelings of wonder and joy and renaissance. How fortunate we are!"
>
> Janet M.

> "I was very much involved with my church before I lost my hearing . . . Gradually, we stopped going because I just couldn't participate very meaningfully. Since [getting my CI], we've started attending a church that has Assistive Listening Devices. It makes such a difference to be able to participate when I can understand every word spoken through a microphone. There are times I'm just overcome with gratitude for the miracle this device can be. Last Sunday, the sermon was on being transformed when change occurs in our lives. Just like a potter sometimes has to crush a pot she's creating to start again, we too sometimes are recreated in something quite different from what we thought we were going to be . . . I took a lot of personal meaning from that message."
>
> Jonathan M.

> "I have always applied my faith in God the same way Arlene wrote about. I prayed for the ability to cope with my hearing loss. I didn't expect to regain my hearing but hoped to find the strength to cope with it. At one point, . . . I was becoming so isolated that I didn't even feel as if I were a part of my own family . . . I prayed so hard to God to help me find a way to deal with it. . . . Lo and behold, I found out about the CI. My prayers have been answered. I agree most of us have a spiritual viewpoint about our CI's, but no one seems to mention it. It is truly a miracle no matter whose eyes it is under."
>
> Nancy D.

Some of my other reports also prompted expressions of hope and understanding:

> "I'm just smiling away and am so happy for you . . . It sounds like heaven. I can't imagine what that would even be like!! But your wonderful posts on how you are doing with your CI gives me so much hope for the future. I'm not afraid anymore of losing the remaining hearing I have. . . ."
>
> Trudy G.

> "Your letters give me the hope that some day I will be able to hear more with less stress . . . I just wanted to thank you for your inspiration and dreams of hope. It does make the light at the end of the tunnel shine a little brighter."
>
> Greg H.

> "I certainly don't take my hearing for granted anymore and I have an even deeper sensitivity to people with hearing losses in social situations. My mother completely withdrew from parties and friends later in life when she lost her hearing. I understand that so much better now."
>
> Lisa C.

Evidently I'm not the first person to discover the art of "manipulated conversations" as this comment shows:

> "When you describe 'manipulating the conversation,' I feel as if we are school girls sharing some sort of secret. So many times people have mentioned that they cannot figure me out, because either I am talking non-stop, or just sitting there and not talking at all. What a colorful personality I must have! Little do they know, what we know, that talking non-stop is the mechanism to make sure we know what the conversation is about, and the silence plain and simple means: no idea what is going on!"
>
> Rachel F.

Even my supermarket stories struck a chord:

> "*I miss those 'Arlene Supermarket Moments.' I never thought I would say that!! I miss hearing the little comments that people make as they stand waiting in line, or listening in on a conversation during a meeting . . . I know exactly what Arlene means when she talks about sitting politely . . . that is me now . . . I am looking forward to being part of the world again . . . I am getting ready to be a "gabber" again!!"*
>
> Caitlin C.

And I guess I'm not the only CI user to rave about root canal, either!:

> "*I had a root canal operation about 6 weeks ago, so I agree with everything you said. The lack of stress this time was awesome.*"
>
> Dave G.

And my August 13 report, where I described behaving "like a real person," brought these responses from other CI users:

> "*Yes, isn't this the best part of it? Having fun like "real people," and laughing, and not having every social situation turn into a stomach-churning moment!!*"
>
> Cindy F.

> "*. . . 'like a real person.' Well, if that doesn't say it all for those of us with CI's, I don't know what will! A sentiment I'm sure most of us share.*"
>
> Linda B.

. . . and this comment from a dear, hard of hearing friend, who understood how I struggled with my hearing loss:

> "*. . . 'like a real person.' Indeed. Welcome back to life, Arlene.*"
>
> Izzy C.

DAY 331
OCTOBER 27

Another annual event has come and gone. Yesterday was the League for the Hard of Hearing's Feast with Famous Faces, another of its major fundraising events, this one earmarked for children's services. It's a grand affair, with over 30 chefs from Manhattan's finest restaurants cooking up appetizer-sized portions of creations from their menus, served by news broadcasters from the television stations. And all of this is accompanied by a live band. You've heard of "ultimate frisbee"? This is Ultimate Cocktail Party.

Last year, I attended this event on the day before my CI surgery. What a difference a year makes! Last year, I barely spoke to anyone, and even then, with great difficulty. I sat, smiled, ate — had a nice time — but. Years before, when my auxiliary microphone worked for me with my hearing aid, I could function, but without that assistance, talking to people in any meaningful way was virtually out of the question.

This year, cool bionic Arlene was having a ball, chatting up a storm with everyone and anyone, and even listening to what people were saying! Gone were the tight, calculating strategies I had developed to survive these affairs. I can't recall doing any calculating last night, now that I mention it. I didn't steer any conversations. I just went with the flow.

I did use my auxiliary microphone. I now have a good idea when I want to use that little gadget and when I don't. I think that hearing people wished they could have had something comparable last night. I saw a lot of strained looks on the faces of normal-hearing people. I was speaking with a friend about how much trouble some hearing people were having, and he replied, "You're a hearing person now." "Nah," I said. "I'm not hearing; I'm bionic." "What's the difference?" he asked. "Bionic means that the music never gets too loud!" I replied.

My own implant surgeon was there as were some other physicians. I couldn't help but feel joy for them, not only for myself. For so many years, they had been forced to concede that there was virtually nothing they could do for those of us with a sensorineural hearing loss. To look at me last night — laughing, chatting, *living* — I felt so good for *them*, that they were now able to perform these miracles.

Towards the end of the evening, there were some short "thank you" speeches — the keynote address given by an 11-year-old boy who has had a CI for eight years. The parents were beaming throughout! They, too, had been touched by the miraculous power of a cochlear implant.

DAY 336
NOVEMBER 1

I've been writing these chronicles for exactly eleven months, and up until now, I was mostly describing feelings and comparing life with my CI to one without. Now I'm finding a different focus: I've gotten used to my CI, and can depend on the level of hearing it gives me. Because of this, I'm starting to branch out, doing things I never would have considered without hearing.

Just last month, I went to a wedding in Ohio by myself. Jeff, my Army penpal from the Persian Gulf War, was getting married and I really wanted to attend. Ira had to go on a business trip to Atlanta, so he couldn't join me. I didn't *have* to go to this wedding. No close family member was involved, so it was not crucial that I be there. It was definitely my choice. Without hearing, the stress of navigating alone wouldn't have been worth it: parking my car, traveling by plane, changing planes, renting a car — all to attend a large social event where I only knew a few people. Of course, if I *had* to do it, I would have. But to *choose* to do this? Not a chance! That would have been torture, not fun.

I'm pleased to report that my Ohio wedding odyssey turned out marvelously well! I was chatting practically non-stop for the entire weekend, often with people I'd never met before. All the travel plans worked out fine. I did miss some of the airline announcements, but I generally knew what was going on. I even got a chance to drive around the cornfields of Ohio by myself, with only a map in hand. How daring! I got semi-lost once and had to yell to a truck driver for directions, but I heard the answer! (It turns out I wasn't lost after all.) I felt like a bird that had been let out of its cage!

Part of this daring had to do with a sense of confidence. I had finally gotten a cellular phone, which was now in my handbag. I didn't feel so vulnerable to the fates, having this little piece of insurance with me. I had a chance to use it too, when I landed back in New York, and had to call the parking garage to pick me up. I had this proud little feeling, "I can do it myself."

Going to that wedding in Ohio is tangible evidence of the confidence this CI has given me. I've also gone to the opera and the movies, and actually enjoyed myself! But even more than that, I feel far more independent, able to go and do things because I'll enjoy them, and not just to prove that I can do them. This has been subtle, taking months to evolve. It took over six months to feel my way with my CI. And now that I've pretty much figured that out, I'm starting to find out who I really am.

What does "who I really am" mean? An example should clarify this. I had an hour-long phone conversation with my 31-year-old niece, Phylisse. We had *never* spoken at length like this before. Our main contact had always been at family gatherings, situations where it looked as if I was involved, but in reality was just part of the scenery. She explained her impressions of me: when the family was talking together, I'd sit there waiting for Ira to tell me what people were saying, and then I'd comment — or as she described it, "deliver a punch line." My whole essence was limited to a punch line! No wonder she didn't know me. How could anyone? Not even me!

I'm discovering my own thoughts, which I'm now free to convey — and also the nuance of what others are saying, so I can respond. I'm learning what it feels like to be free to think without being burdened by the struggle to hear. This wasn't apparent to me in the first few months of CI "wonder," exactly what it means to be able to communicate with ease. I was too preoccupied with the mechanics, the raw ability to hear. Now I'm ready to appreciate the subtleties of human communication and how it shapes our behavior and personality.

I'm finding out that I have a lot to say! (Maybe because I have to make up for thirty years of going deaf!) I've never felt this sort of freedom before, free to be me! This, too, is part of the progression of being able to hear again. I don't think it's possible to be thrust back into the world of sound and not take some time to adjust. It's like turning the lights on in the middle of the night; it takes a while for the eyes to see clearly again. Likewise, it has taken me time first to adjust to the sounds, and now to the impact of it all.

DAY 339
NOVEMBER 4

Yesterday was Election Day and some "ghosts" surfaced again. As I went to vote, as I'd done in the same location for the last 15 years, I again wondered if I would be able to hear the poll workers. I always hated going there because they would invariably start chatting, and I would consciously hope that no one would talk to me. Yesterday, I finally understood them. The woman behind "the book" asked for my name, told me "Yes, I thought you were in the R's," told me where to sign, and then where to sign again. I got every word! I walked out of there feeling the same way I have been feeling this past year — no sweat, no work, no struggle. I felt "light," and I still can't get over how something that had been so stressful without hearing was a total "non-event" with my CI!

From there I went to my eye doctor to see if I needed new reading glasses. Those eye exams had always been stressful because I'd have to watch the doctor for instructions and then read the eye charts, switching back and forth between lipreading and chart-reading. Yesterday — *voila!* — I didn't have to look at the doctor at all to understand his instructions. Again, what used to be such work when I couldn't hear was ridiculously simple now.

Comments keep trickling in, and someone wondered if there were any negative effects from my CI on family members. "Are you never impatient with Ira, or he with you?," they wanted to know. That was a funny question because the answer is that impatience was the norm when I *couldn't* hear. In the car, for example, the only way Ira and I could communicate was if I was looking at him. But sometimes something would catch my eye out the window, so I did not always want to "pay attention." This produced impatience and frustration for both of us. Now that I can hear him without looking, this problem no longer exists.

This question prompted me to ask Ira if he had any thoughts of his own about my hearing again, in addition to the ease of communication. Ira pointed out that he no longer worries about me during the day when I'm on my own. He always worried about my getting lost, or needing help, and not being able to fend for myself. He also said that it was a relief not having me so stressed out all the time — not only smiling more, but no longer waking up at night crying. Yes, he's right. I used to wake up crying practically every night, overwhelmed and worried about how I would get through the next day. I still wake up with thoughts on my mind, but I stopped crying when I got my CI. The stress that was producing those tears is gone. So finally, Ira is able to get through the night stress-free too. Again, we sometimes overlook the impact hearing loss has on others, especially those closest to us.

DAY 347
NOVEMBER 12

This is a three-part story, all intertwined, beginning with the special Yizkor (memorial) service this past Yom Kippur. This was my second time "saying Yizkor" for my father, who had passed away a year and a half ago. Last year, with hardly any hearing to follow the service, I sat mostly in quiet meditation. This year, with my CI and the infrared listening system in my synagogue, I was hearing astonishingly well. The Rabbi began the service by asking us first to close our eyes. "Close my eyes?" I thought. My gut reaction was that I couldn't do that. How would I be sure to hear it all with no visual cues? I had never participated in anything with my eyes closed — no yoga classes, relaxation sessions, meditation. I was always an "eyes open" person. But this was different, and I was different now too. I took a huge leap of faith and closed my eyes.

The Rabbi continued, asking us to concentrate on one of our departed loved ones, and then to imagine them sitting next to us. "Tell them what you'd like them to know," he said. And I could do that! I could sit there understanding the Rabbi's every word, even with my eyes closed. As instructed, I had a short discussion with my father. I told him that I could hear again! And also that we were taking good care of my mother, who has Alzheimer's. It felt good to do this and I felt like part of the congregation, as well as feeling closer to my father. The service resumed in the usual manner — eyes open — reading from the text. But the experience stayed with me. I did something I couldn't have done last year, and it made an impression on me.

A few weeks later — and this is Part II of the story — I received a Relay call. I asked immediately which way this call was going — was I the hearing person or the deaf person? I didn't know if someone was unaware of my new telephone skills, since my phone number is often given with a "Voice/TTY" suffix. It turned out that it was a call from someone who was about to have CI surgery. She had gotten my name and number from a mutual friend. I was the hearing party in this Relay call. This was my third time doing this, and let me tell you, I can appreciate a *lot* more what hearing callers have to put up with when using Relay! I knew to speak slowly, and this Relay operator was pretty good about getting it all down without asking me to repeat. The woman calling had many questions about the CI, good ones that only another CI user could answer. I've always felt a personal obligation to take my time with people's CI questions. I know firsthand how important this whole CI process is. I spent a lot of time on the phone with her, missing my favorite tv program, "Jeopardy," in the process. Waiting for the operator to type my words, I could hear the click-clicking of the keys and then the voiced response. I knew how to end Relay calls graciously, without seeming to hang up abruptly. The trick that I had used, even as a deaf user, was to announce that I was going to say "Good-bye," which served as a prompt for the other person to say "good-bye" too. I felt good about that call even though it took so long.

Part III of the story happened just a few days later. I had a dream that my father called me by Relay and that I was the hearing person! But my father wasn't using Voice Carryover. He had the Relay Operator voice the call for him, even though it was a female operator. (So much for the idea that God is a He!) I could hear everything perfectly. Sure, it was only a dream, and you'd figure that there's no reason not to hear in a dream, but that was never the case. From the very beginnings of my hearing loss, 30 years ago, my dream hearing always reflected my actual hearing. I remember having my first hard of hearing dream, having to ask "WHAT," and thinking when I awoke, "Don't I even get a break in my dreams?" This dream was significant because I didn't ask "WHAT?" at all. My brain had evidently made the transition — had, in effect, decided that I had good enough hearing now to pass for hearing — at least in my dreams!

In this dream, I asked my father why he was calling me by Relay, and he replied that it was a free service where he was calling from. He told me that he was no longer living with my mother, and that he had taken an apartment in Washington Township. (My synagogue is in Washington Township!) He wanted to see my mother, so I told him I would take him to visit her. We met and went to see her together, in a lovely grassy lawn area where she was sitting on a settee shaded from the sun by a canopy. And then I woke up. It took me a moment to orient myself and realize that my father was not really alive. Everything had seemed so real!

I am still learning how much we absorb with our hearing. The directions of the Rabbi in the synagogue, the voices of the women on Relay (both caller and operator.) These voices literally touched my soul. What power the sense of hearing has — and what power this CI has, even when it is sitting on the night table by my bed, switched off.

DAY 352
NOVEMBER 17

I just spent a few days away from home and that has given me some fresh perspectives on how I function now with my CI. I'm still "hard of hearing" but not in the same way I was with a hearing aid. I hear so well, so often, that I've developed a new behavior pattern: I don't watch people's faces anymore — maybe in my peripheral vision, but not intensely. My confidence in being able to catch what is being said, without that piercing gaze, has produced this behavior. But I don't get everything all the time, so I'll ask for a repeat if I miss something, this time paying attention, and that's been working pretty well for me. This seems to be "what I do," a subtle blend of hearing, coping skills, lipreading and low stress casual behavior.

In moderate noise, I'll switch to my noise program or turn down the sensitivity setting, and know that I'll have to watch (i.e. do some lipreading). Variables of noise intensity and people's voices determine how much watching I have to do to augment what I'm hearing. I've found that there is a certain degree of lipreading that my brain refuses to do anymore and it nudges me to put on my auxiliary mic. It likes sound and knows where to get it in a (noisy) pinch.

Some voices are easier for me to hear, but I've found no rhyme or reason to this. I was in the supermarket recently, having a hard time understanding the cashier, even with full view of her face — yet the person at my side told me what she said, and I understood *her* without even looking! Hit or miss!

I've been in a few situations where the background noise has been a problem, usually a competing conversation nearby. When that happens, I'll mention to the person I'm speaking with that I have a hearing problem. The funny thing is, I have no negative emotions attached to that declaration anymore. It used to be that mentioning my hearing loss was a prologue to my tale of woe. But now — wow! — I have a hearing loss that sometimes gets in the way of smooth communications, but look, I'm really deaf, so it's absolutely amazing for me to be hearing as much as I do!

We attended a show in my in-laws' condominium in Florida, an annual rite for the past 23 years. One of the most frustrating experiences for me has been sitting in an audience where everyone is convulsed with laughter — except me — because I couldn't hear the comedian well enough to understand what was so funny. For all those years, I politely sat there for the obligatory hour. I couldn't *not* go. The whole family was there, but I definitely couldn't enjoy myself either — 23 years of this.

This year was the first time in memory that I could hear the comedian. I was sitting in the second row, he had a microphone, and I got it all. I finally got to laugh with everyone else! And the old Borscht Belt jokes everyone knows? They were all fresh to me, as if I had been born yesterday.

DAY 355
NOVEMBER 20

Not to dwell on the negatives of this CI, but as I gain more experience with this device, there are definitely some "inconveniences." Aside from the problems of listening in noise, there are the physical limitations — like not being able to get it wet. I have to take off the external components to go swimming or take a shower, so those are activities that I have to do "deaf." That forces me to make social decisions, too, like choosing between swimming OR hearing, since I can't do both at the same time.

I also have to take my CI off at night, so I'm deaf then too. All the alerting devices that I used before, I still need. I have a strobe visual alert in my bedroom for the phone, doorbell, and fire alarm, and I have a vibrator to put under the mattress which is also connected to this system. That's one reason that no matter how well I hear with my CI, I can't forget that I'm deaf — not for long anyway — because I'm deaf every night. It's *very* quiet at night. Well, *almost* quiet. I still have tinnitus, a constant ringing in my ears, that I have always had. (I remember, as a child, thinking that I could "hear silence.") I barely notice it now when my CI is on, but when it's off, there it is again!

I'm not sure if this is a negative, but now my communications come in uncensored — for better or worse. I'm learning that much of the dialogue that had reached me in the past had been "cleaned up" or filtered. It seems that it had taken so much effort to have a conversation with me, I was spared trivia, sarcasm, profanity and similar tidbits that were deemed "not important" enough to convey to me. Even when some of these realities of life did slip through, they would never be repeated if I missed them the first time, and then had to ask "What?" Any indiscretion or inelegance would immediately be retracted if given a second chance. This held true for Relay calls as well. My sister said it was like "having your mother watching." People were always on their best behavior.

I'm learning that the world isn't quite as genteel as it was when communication with me was "by invitation only." I don't think this is necessarily bad — or good. It's REAL. With so much more information coming my way, I'm learning there are many dimensions to people and situations. The world is a lot more colorful when you can hear the witticisms and incidental remarks as well as what is "important," and this is in addition to the nuances of the speech itself. It just surprised me a little to see *everyone* in greater depth. I hadn't anticipated that.

DAY 365
NOVEMBER 30

I was rushing out the door the other day when I heard the phone ring. Arms full, I ran back into the kitchen, dumped the load I was carrying onto the table, and dashed for the phone. I reached with my right hand, picked up the receiver and held it up to my right ear, saying "hello." As soon as that receiver reached my head — "OY! I forgot! I'm deaf!" I quickly transferred the receiver to my left hand and held it up to the head mic of my CI. Had I really convinced myself that I'm now a hearing person? How could I have forgotten that I need to use the telephone with my CI mic? I'll leave the explanations to the armchair psychologists.

This past weekend we went with friends to the Jackson Pollock exhibit at the Museum of Modern Art. This was the first time I had an opportunity to take a museum audio tape tour since getting my CI. This tape tour was essential for viewing the exhibit because there was no way that I could begin to appreciate Jackson Pollock's splatters without some help. My comments on the exhibit will have to wait for a different forum, but the hearing experience, I can describe.

My friends were going to be following the tape tour too, and I had absolutely no hesitation to do just what everyone else was doing. I could, and I knew I could. I didn't have to ask for the transcript, which I'd done in the past. I did forego the headphones, which I didn't need, since I don't really have "ears" anymore. I just plugged my patch cord from cassette recorder to speech processor, and followed the instructions and dialogue, just like everyone else there in that crowded exhibit space.

One of the highlights of this tour was a jazz interlude played at one of the gallery displays. I followed the instructions on the tape, which told me to listen to the jazz and observe yet another splattered "masterpiece." There was an older gentleman, obviously up to the same portion of the tape, bobbing his head in time to the music as he gazed at the painting. I gave him a knowing smile as I too bobbed in time to the music. He looked back at me, and looked again — and I realized that he must have been wondering why I was bobbing when I had no headphones on! I didn't say a word. I'm sure he's still wondering!

Thanksgiving Weekend has just passed and it was a lot different from last year. I expected Thanksgiving would be the crowning touch of a year of awakening and revelations — and it was. Family gatherings are no longer trying experiences, so this Thanksgiving was relaxing and enjoyable, just as I thought it would be. I made a special toast — to appreciate how far I'd come from Thanksgivings of years past. I reflected on how difficult it had been for me when I couldn't follow the free flow of conversation, and how warm and wonderful when I could.

Last year, I had great expectations, and this year they were realities. I remember last Thanksgiving wondering if I would really be able to hear again. The idea seemed too fantastic, even though I knew other people who had experienced it. I even wondered if I would remember how to hear. It all seemed too much to hope for. Listening and reading about others expressing thanks for their own CI's at Thanksgiving last year, I had hope, but doubts. Could this really happen to me? Now I know. Yes, it can — and yes, it has.

DAY 369
DECEMBER 4

I had my one-year evaluation and mapping yesterday, a rite of passage in this CI journey. There were no surprises. I knew how I was doing — no numbers or tests really mattered to me. As I sat there reciting word lists and sentences, I felt once again that it was my speech processor being tested and not my hearing. For the curious, I could repeat almost 100% of the sentences in quiet and in moderate noise, and almost 80% of single syllable words. I even had an audiogram done, which tested the pure tone sounds I could hear, and showed that I performed as someone with a mild hearing loss. It was funny to see an audiogram workup sheet for this faux hearing. It was like building cities on the ashes of what had come before — my own true hearing, which is nil. So congratulations are in order to the wizards at Advanced Bionics Corporation, makers of my Clarion device — and, of course, to my surgeon, Dr. Ronald Hoffman, and my audiologist, Betsy Bromberg. They passed my faux hearing test with flying colors!

I celebrated my actual one-year anniversary on December 1, by inviting a Brownie Girl Scout troop of 15 girls to my house to view my special collection of Girl Scout and Brownie dolls. I would never have attempted this *sans* hearing, so it was a very fitting way to mark one year with my implant. I had a great time, chatting with the girls. I didn't catch everything, of course, but that didn't matter. I knew I could if they all quieted down. They were working on an "Etiquette" badge, so when our session was over, I had each of them shake my hand and say, "Thank you. It was nice to meet you." I responded to each and every girl, and I loved hearing all their little voices. The leader, a friend of mine, reported back to me that one of the girls had told her, "I think that lady really liked me. She kept looking at me and smiling." That little girl had it right, and must have sensed something special going on. The wonder is still there, the delight at being able to do things, hear things long missing from my life.

I don't think this wonder is going to fade either. About a dozen times a day, I'm reminded how my behavior is different because I can hear. I welcome human contact. I no longer walk through the day hoping that no one will speak to me. I'm a part of the world around me, not isolated in my silence or confined to my own thoughts.

I know that my hearing is not normal and I know that I'm still really deaf, even though I'm masquerading as a hearing person, albeit one with a mild hearing loss. The funny thing is that I tend to feel a bit sorry for hearing people, who take their normal hearing for granted. They'll never understand the special joy and wonder that I experience each and every day of being able to hear again.

And that is where I will end these chronicles. It has been a year since I began reporting my CI exploits. I had only intended to write about my initial hookup. But the comments kept flowing in, literally from all over the globe, to please keep writing about my experiences. From those with hearing, and those without, friends and family, professionals in the field, those comments kept me writing. I think you now have a good idea what this cochlear implant is all about.

My mother taught me that it is wise to end a party while everyone is still enjoying themselves. And my grandmother's words about "not overstaying one's welcome" come to mind as well. It's been a pleasure sharing my story with you. And now comes the hardest part — the "happily ever after." My best wishes to you all.

> "*How fortunate [we are] that you have been celebrating [with us] all year, shining an ever clear, bright light on lingering dark corners of doubt and despair, and repeatedly bringing us back to the heart of the CI experience: the transformation — swift and dramatic for some, slow and quiet for others — from isolation to growing engagement or re-engagement with our fellow human beings and with hitherto unknown worlds.*
>
> *No man, woman or child is an "island," however self-contained they may appear to be. Your wonderful string of posts, tossed like shiny pebbles on the great wide ocean, have created waves of recognition upon our shores. We've caught your treasures in the 'Net' and savored the sweetness of your liberation and the joy of your discoveries.*"

Anne-Marie L. (CI user)

HOW A COCHLEAR IMPLANT WORKS

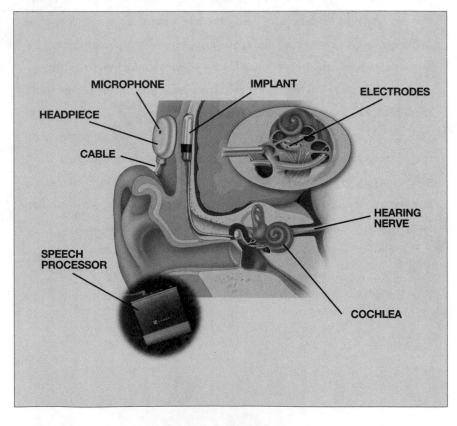

Illustration courtesy of Advanced Bionics Corporation.

Sound waves enter the **MICROPHONE** located in the **HEADPIECE** and are converted into an electrical signal. The **HEADPIECE** is held on by magnets.

This signal is sent to the **SPEECH PROCESSOR** via the thin **CABLE** that connects the **HEADPIECE** to the **SPEECH PROCESSOR**.

The **SPEECH PROCESSOR** converts the electrical signal into a distinctive digital code which is programmed specifically to maximize each individual's sound and speech understanding.

Once processed, the electrically coded signal is sent back up the thin **CABLE** to the **HEADPIECE** and is transmitted through the scalp via radio waves to the **IMPLANT**.

The **IMPLANT** decodes the signal and delivers it to the array of **ELECTRODES** positioned deep within the **COCHLEA**.

The **ELECTRODES** bypass the damaged hair cells and directly stimulate the **HEARING NERVE** fibers within the **COCHLEA**.

Stimulation of the **HEARING NERVE** fibers causes electrical impulses to be delivered to the brain where they are interpreted as sound.

INDEX